SILENCE
EQUALS
SUICIDE

Love Yourself to Live

Caroline
I am so glad we crossed
paths! Please stay in
touch!
♥ / *[signature]*

SILENCE EQUALS SUICIDE

Love Yourself to Live

Jamie Ryser

Printed in the United States of America.
ISBN-13: 979-8-9898625-0-4 Paperback
979-8-9898625-1-1 Hardcover
979-8-9898625-2-8 eBook
LCCN: Applied for

Jamie Ryser Publishing
Palm Bay, Florida

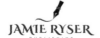

JAMIE RYSER
PUBLISHING

To my beautiful children Ryker and Kambria. My love for you is unconditional and permanent. Thank you for teaching me how to be a better person, babies. To my family, your love carried me through the darkness and helped teach me to love myself. To my ride or dies, thank you for teaching me not everyone leaves. I love you all.

Table of Contents

Introduction

Approximately 1.7 million adults attempted suicide in 2021, of those 1.7 million attempts 48,183 Americans died by suicide.[1]

So, what happens after they try? Why aren't we talking about the continued pain of multiple attempts? Someone attempts to take their life once, and then what? Are they healed? I think the fuck not. Life is hard, and by not talking about suicide, society creates a stigma around attempted suicide, wondering why this person isn't healed or "fixed."

This book is meant to start conversations! Do you struggle with the darkness? Do you feel like a burden? Do you have tools that help you? How has suicide impacted your life? I am not afraid to talk about my darkness because I have tools that help me not wind up on that bathroom floor again.

By reading this book, I hope it gives you the courage to talk about your darkness. Growth doesn't come through silence, talking about the dark shit is how we help. I have learned these

---

[1] *"Suicide Statistics." American Foundation for Suicide Prevention*

skills through actually talking about the dark shit! People have taught me different things to pull myself through because I was willing to ask for help and discuss it.

As I wrote this book I found immense healing. The tools I use, the lessons I learned, all helped me begin my spiritual journey. I hope this book helps you find healing too. Mark it up, dog ear the corners, write in it. This is your healing journey. There are certain tools that require you to write. I recommend having a journal you use as you read. This is your journey now. Make it your own and expand your tools to better your mental health. You deserve a beautiful, radiant life, so if you are here reading this book, welcome! I applaud you for taking the first step to choosing you, and hope you have a journey of healing, peace, and love.

Everyone deserves a toolbelt full of various coping skills and tools. There must be a safe place to talk about that darkness to grow your skills. We can create that safe space. Silence equals suicide. Read on if you refuse to stay silent anymore!

Chapter 1

The Journey Begins Friends

In September 2022, I sat on the bathroom floor after attempting suicide, crying as my husband held me.

There weren't sirens or flashing lights. It was intimate; just two people fighting for different things. It was my sweet husband wrestling the dog grooming shears out of my hands as blood pooled on the floor from my wrists being sliced up the vein.

When you have a doctorate in all nineteen seasons of *Grey's Anatomy*, you know how to kill yourself by slitting your wrists.

It was fall in beautiful Wyoming. The skies were the perfect blue, leaves were falling, and I was in my home, nestled in some mountains. But, my mental health didn't allow me to see the beauty all around me, I was trapped in my darkness.

The darkness amplifies little difficulties, making them seem more immense and unbearable.

The seemingly small things added up one day, and I couldn't do it anymore. I didn't write a note; I was past that. My husband knew of the ways I felt inadequate. He knew I thought I was a burden instead of a blessing. So, why write a note?

I had just fired a horse trainer who was a potential business partner and I felt mentally exhausted. I just wanted to rest permanently. We put the kids down for a nap, my husband started farm work, and I went into the bathroom with my dog grooming shears. Good shears are expensive and slice through the skin like a hot knife to butter.

I remember the cold tile as I sat between the bathtub and shower, pleading to the Universe that my existence wouldn't be missed. I was so fucking tired, I just wanted to sleep. So, I sliced my arm upwards, following the vein. The cut hurt, but not as bad as the constant ache of inadequacy I felt.

I truly believed I would be doing everyone a favor. The thing with suicide is, as selfish of an act as it may seem, I truly believed that my children and those who loved me would be better off without me. We create our reality, and that was mine. I knew it would hurt them, but in the long run, my self-worth was so low that I genuinely believed they would heal and the hurt my existence caused would outweigh the pain of losing me.

Everyone talks about the pain, but all I remember was exhaustion. I wanted to sleep. That permanent sleep never came because the Universe wasn't ready for me to be done. My husband decided to come in and check on me because he knew firing a friend had been hard. His timing saved my life.

Everything seemed to move in slow motion. He unlocked the door and plowed in. He saw me curled in a ball, bleeding on the floor with the shears in my hand. Immediately he went straight for the shears and tore them out of my hands. I did my best to fight him, screaming for him to leave me alone.

I saw his devastation as tears streamed down his face. My husband doesn't cry easily, so my heart broke to see his tears. I caused that pain, but thought I was doing him a favor.

My husband pulled me onto his lap, and the cold from the tile was replaced with the warmth of his body. He held towels against my wrists. The one person who saw all of me was begging me to fight.

At that moment, on the floor, my heart broke as he held me *because I was still there*. My attempt "failed." Again. I was devastated; because, in my mind, his saving me was creating more of a burden than just letting me go.

"Just fucking let me go!" I pleaded through my sobs as he clung to me, holding the blood-soaked towels to my wrists. He refused to let me go. He fought for me when I couldn't fight for myself. He just held me, holding the towels and repeatedly saying he was there.

The good moments shape you, but the challenging moments define you. In this moment of devastation, we were both changed. My husband has always seen me in the light of love, whereas I tend to see flaws and imperfections.

That is why this book has become so important to me. It is me choosing to see myself through the Divine lens of love. You have to choose to fill your cup because as much love as my husband has for me, he can't fill my cup. Every day it takes work. It is hard to choose to fill your cup, but who will if you don't? My husband can hold me through my tears but can't feed my soul.

The good moments shape you, but the challenging moments define you.

Eventually, the blood and tears stopped. But, that "failed" attempt changed my life. It wasn't my first attempt, it was my second of three attempts. I had one other attempt after the shears on the bathroom floor. My second attempt is what began the true healing journey. I got help in the way that I needed it, but that doesn't mean my desire to not exist just ceased. But again, the second attempt was the most enlightening one for my soul. Healing is a journey, not a destination.

After the first attempt, I had been institutionalized in the hospital and didn't want to be again. The hospital didn't help me. I needed true healing, not meds and locked doors. We spent the next two days brainstorming where I could go to get help and healing.

Trying to figure out where I wanted to go was like ripping teeth from my mouth. I didn't want to go anywhere. Not existing sounded easier; I was fucking exhausted. I grew up with the expectation that I was supposed to be perfect. I expected perfection from myself, and anything less than that was not enough. Striving for perfection in an imperfect world is exhausting, which is why not existing felt like it would've been better. If I can't be perfect, I might as well not exist. I thought I needed out.

Knowing that healing isn't linear or something that happens overnight is critical to the healing journey. I needed compassion for myself. I needed a place where I could find compassion instead of hatred within.

What I needed was to connect to my Divine and find true healing. Attempted suicide permanently altered my life because healing becomes necessary only when we are completely broken.

My story is about understanding that healing is possible, but just like with alcohol and drugs, suicidal ideation is something that the "user" has to learn how to live through. Days come when my thoughts go to suicide, but I choose to fight those thoughts. I honestly don't know if suicide will ever not pop into my head, but my acquired skills have taught me to see myself through the lens of the infinite love of the Universe.

I am no longer afraid to talk about suicide because people die of this disease when we stay silent. The less we talk about suicide, the more people we will find on their bathroom floors dying.

Chapter 2

Destined Disney Friend

Two weeks before my suicide attempt, I was on a girls' trip to Disneyland. Being the Disney fanatic I am, I was in charge of the Genie+ pass and ensuring we had our Lightning Lanes all set. Excited to get to Disney, I grabbed my portable charger but forgot the cord. We weren't even halfway through our day, and my phone was already at 13% battery. We had to use my phone for the passes. I kept looking for people I could ask to use their cords and even used one person's cord for about 45 seconds before she got on the ride.

After I rode It's A Small World, I accepted the fact that I would have to buy a cord so I could continue using our Lightning Lanes. I also accepted that aside from the annoying repetitive song, It's A Small World is beautiful because it highlights the different countries, ethnicities, and the diverse world we live in. It truly is a small world because we are Divine beings connected through the infinite love of the Universe.

By the ride exit, there was a little gift shop. I had been hunting to find my kids a souvenir, but I found something priceless. I was looking at the Rapunzel pins debating on which one to add to my collection, when I heard a woman ask the cast member (that is what they call employees), "I know this is a long shot, but is there a place that I can plug my charger in for my phone?" What a small world that someone would need a place to charge their phone, and I happened to have one!

An important fact about me is that I am not afraid of people. This has been a useful skill throughout my life. I said, "Okay, this might be super weird, but I brought my portable charger and forgot the cord, so if you want to let me use your cord, I will let you use my portable charger."

This chick was around 5'1 with perfect hair, the cutest leopard print Minnie Mouse ears, and the cutest Mickey shirt that I had been eyeballing all day at the gift shops! She carried herself with confidence and energy, which attracted people to her like Disney fans are attracted to their favorite ride. Within thirty seconds, I knew I wanted her in my friend circle. Her name was Jessi, and it was like Walt held her hand and walked her over to me to introduce us. It was indeed a destined Disney friendship.

She said yes to sharing her cord and tagged along with us for the rest of the evening. Our acquaintanceship quickly snowballed into a beautiful friendship, and fast-forward to now, I would say that Jessi is one of my soulmates. I don't mean soulmate in that I-am-going-to-marry-her type of way, but in the way that my soul knows her. We met at a magical place and have continued to bring light and love into each other's life. She is one of my best friends and has taught me more about connecting to the Universe than I ever thought possible.

Less than two weeks after meeting her, I found myself on the bathroom floor after my attempted suicide. My husband told me I was going to a hospital or an inpatient care system. I researched various places, but my mind kept telling me to call Jessi and ask her about her place. Jessi didn't know the severity of my depression, and no one besides my family knew I had just attempted to end my life. So, I called her, and the next night, I was sleeping at Estuary.

Estuary is a retreat for your body and soul to find healing. It is where you can step away from the world and into a sanctioned space meant for personal healing and Divine growth.

Jessi had an entire team working endlessly to get things ready for me, she even had pictures of my kids and nods to Disney in my room. Walking into my room, I realized that I am not in this life alone and that every interaction matters. I had people fighting for me to stay, who I didn't even know were in my corner.

Jessi even picked me up wearing her Minnie Mouse ears! Here was this beautiful woman I had only known for two weeks picking me up from the airport, planning an entire seven-day retreat, and showing up for me simply because she loved me. Jessi wanted to be there for me. She saw a Divine Being and was willing to drop everything to ensure I was okay.

The Universe has a plan. I was in a dark place and had tunnel vision that gave me one option. Suicide. That attempt failed because the Universe knew I needed to meet Jessi and experience Estuary.

The Universe helped everything fall into place because I was finally ready to embrace personal healing. I was financially able to go to Estuary. Jessi's team prepped for me in less than 24 hours, my husband could be with the kids, and a million other things fell into place so I could begin my healing.

Estuary was a retreat center, focused on various types of healing. At Estuary, we did a lot of meditation, connecting with nature by swimming in the river, walking through the woods, getting body painted and doing power photo shoots, EDMR therapy, one-on-one life coaching sessions, saltwater tank healing meditations, journal sessions, and other healing activities. The focus was on finding yourself and connecting your soul to the Divine.

There was a lot of silence at Estuary. It was a time when I was solely focused on my healing and discovering why my soul was in so much pain.

I finally took time to reflect inwardly to discover who I was, and what my soul needed.

I learned that not everyone has to go to Estuary to achieve healing. There are tools we all can utilize to experience immense healing and know our Divine selves.

You must dig to the root of the healing and ask yourself: what hurt have you suppressed so deeply? I am not a doctor, so in no way am I giving medical advice. Throughout my healing journey, I have learned my medicine was a band-aid covering what I was feeling. Lexapro could only do so much for me when I hated myself. If I didn't begin to heal my soul, no medicinal dosage would help my depression. I had tried for years, seen so many doctors, and spent so much money, but I needed true healing and no Western medicine doctor was able to give that to me.

Not everyone has the opportunity to go to Estuary, or spend a bunch of money on medications. But there are tools throughout this book that I hope helps heal a little of your soul. In writing this book, I discovered myself. There are so many ways we can connect with the Universe, and as we strive to do that in every day we will find growth with every sunset.

As we get to know our divine purpose, and the abundant power the Universe has we find a connection that takes us beyond just our day to day life. Recognizing that the Universe is an infinite source of love gives you the ability to see yourself as a Divine being. Being a Divine being means your perspective is beyond the day to day life. Creating a life of hope and light takes time. You have to prioritize your peace. But as you do little things throughout the day you will see yourself with an infinite love and with unlimited power.

You can achieve anything you put your mind to, even if you feel stuck. Creating your Estuary will take time, because again, it is a state of mind. There is a corner in my room that I have blessed, and only put things that strengthen my spiritual growth there. It is where I meditate, journal, read self-help books, and connect to my Divine. This safe space I have created allows me to get to know myself on a spiritual connection, I see myself as the powerful being I am whenever I am in this corner.

Knowing our Divine selves means we recreate ourselves every day through focusing our intentions on the Universe. We live on a higher vibration of love and light, being intentional in our thoughts and actions, and using discernment in making Higher Choices for ourselves.

French Philosopher Pierre Teilhard de Chardin said, "We are not human beings having a spiritual experience; we are spiritual beings having a human experience." Knowing your Divine self is recognizing that you are a spiritual being created by an essence of love. The Universe is full of infinite and abundant love, and your human experience can be phenomenal as you learn tools to heal.

The Universe has our back. You just have to take the first step to begin healing. You are worthy of finally seeing yourself through the Divine lens of infinite, unconditional love. You may feel like your only option is suicide, but I promise the Universe has a plan. I know the darkness is suffocating. It buries you.

You have to actively move through the darkness to experience light. Trusting that the Universe is an essence of love and that you can live on a higher vibration of joy is scary. But trust that you will find light amongst the darkness. Darkness can't reside where light is. Choose today to commit to creating your own Estuary. This book can be a guide to help you connect to the Divine.

Lower energies can't exist among high energies. If you live your life on a higher vibration, then no outside sources can remove you from that higher vibration. High energy converts low energy. Think about it for a minute. When you are with someone who has an energy of love, how does that make you feel? Have you ever been with someone who just feels good to be around? It raises your vibration. Your energy levels are raised.

You can create that same energy for yourself. This book is all about being active in our healing. You must choose to raise your vibrational state of living. Living with depression and anxiety sometimes feels suffocating. There have been times when I felt like the weight of the world was suffocating me.

But as I choose daily to create a space of peace within myself. Each morning when I first wake up, I choose peace. I choose to feel the vibrations I felt at Estuary. Estuary has become a state of mind, not a physical place. You don't have to go to a physical place to find healing; healing starts here. Right now. Let's go, babe. I got you!

Chapter 3

There Is Beauty In The Grey

S tepping into acceptance of our Divine selves is all about trusting the process! Recently, I started painting, and trusting the process has become the key to my art. The style of painting I do is called Dutch pouring. This process seems simple, but takes various tools and an understanding of manipulating the paint. You must be in control enough to guide the paint but release control enough to trust when to let it maneuver independently.

I have acrylic paint, and I pour it directly onto the canvas. I then manipulate the paint using a blow dryer, straw, or by tipping the canvas. The paint is moved based on the manipulation given. I love this art style because you genuinely never know the result, regardless of how hard you try to control it. I can have an idea, but it is always different than intended.

Healing comes when we trust that we are the canvas and the Universe is creating a spectacular piece of art. We are held by hands that create infinite beauty.

I have completed several canvases, and each one is unique but beautiful. There was one specific painting where I was nervous it would turn out ugly. Through the painting process, it became muddled, and I thought I added too many colors together. It almost had a grey look. The more I manipulated the air, the more spread out the colors became.

I wanted to throw away that canvas and redo it before completion. I chose to trust the process; I chose to trust that the result would be something beautiful.

Essentially, I layer the colors, and as the air moves them around, various colors are revealed. So, though it looked like a chaotic mess, the expansion of the colors was revealing, and it was genuinely beautiful.

This same concept applies to life. I didn't know that Estuary would change my life. The process to get there seemed like an ugly, muddled mess. Trying to end my life seemed messy, but there was a Divine manipulation that I was unaware of. There was a reason I survived. My existence adds value, and my presence is necessary.

Before you try to end your life, end the life you are living. What in your life is creating the grey muddled mess? Is it your job, your habits, or your environment? Do you need to move across the country? What do you need to kill, besides yourself, to allow colors to come through?

There is a reason that YOU are here, darlin'! Your existence adds value, and your presence is necessary. Even if you don't see your value, there is a purpose to you being here. No one can tell you your purpose, or give it to you. You need to discover it for yourself. Living authentically to ourselves is key to finding our purpose. What in your life is keeping you from living life to the fullest?

When our lives seem like a chaotic mess of grey, we may have to trust that the individual colors have yet to be uncovered. You are a divine piece of art. You are beautiful regardless of the mess you may find yourself in.

There is beauty in the grey. My grey became my greatest gift. Because of my grey, my eyes were finally opened to Divine healing. A Divine source created you, full of infinite and unconditional love.

I recognize that I am a Divine being, but seeing that in my day-to-day life takes a conscious effort. Focusing on the Divine is acting in mindfulness. Being mindful means we are present in the moment.

There is an activity I like to do when I feel stuck and against the Universe. This is called the "yes" activity. This is where I say yes to every emotion and thought that comes up. We embrace the grey by accepting what comes our way.

If sadness comes up, I lean into that and figure out why I am feeling those feelings. I say yes to the sadness coming up, I don't avoid it like I used to. I trust that the Universe had a reason for that emotion to pop up. Me saying yes to the feelings could look like crying, actually letting the tears go, instead of taking deep breaths to force them away.

The more we resist, the more things persist. By saying yes to the emotions, instead of suppressing them, I allow inner healing to take place. My "Bonus Mom" or Step Mom Lisa recently told me that I can either feel the pain now, or I can feel it later. Either way, I am going to feel it because it will come up in other ways. She said it is okay not to feel it right now, you can choose not to, but there will be a time when you will have to acknowledge your feelings.

I have an exercise for you. If you have feelings that you are suppressing because you fear the pain of feeling them, when you are ready give yourself 90 seconds. Set a timer, and feel those feelings. Every tear, and scream, and sorrow. Feel them. Begin by saying "I am present in the moment by choosing to feel safe in my feelings and trusting that the Universe is an abundant force of love."

As you work through the emotions, don't shove any down or push them away. You can do it for 90 seconds. I genuinely believe that by sitting in the feelings, you can finally allow yourself to move through them. When we allow ourselves to feel what we have ignored, we can begin healing by accepting and acknowledging. Acknowledge the feeling, sit in it. Again, don't ignore the pain. You must feel the pain to feel the peace.

The Universe will not leave you in a muddled mess. You will find growth in every experience if your perspective is open. Lotus flowers are a lot like life. These flowers thrive under challenging environments but emerge from murky depths. They grow in muddy water. We are Lotus flowers, and through our Divine growth, beauty will arise.

You must feel the pain to feel the peace.

When we accept our Divine selves, we know life is limitless. There is no cap on success, happiness, and love. If we are constantly feeding into the darkness and negativity, that is what we will see. As we choose growth, we will see growth.

Daily, take time to see and truly feel the feelings you have. I like to put my hand over my heart, or tap my chest and say the feelings that I am experiencing. "Sadness, trapped, darkness, afraid, alone, not worthy, failure, etc." whatever I am feeling, I name. As you name the feelings you take away their power and control over you.

I was going on a walk with my kiddos because my anxiety and depression was starting to overwhelm me. As we were walking, I started naming my feelings. As I named them, I took away the power and hold they had over me. I didn't allow my emotions to control me, because I didn't fear them. I used to fear feelings. My fear in feelings would show up by me running away from them and burying them. I was actively choosing fear instead of love, because I was burying hard emotions.

I would put an emotion in a box and hide it away in the darkest crevices of my mind. By choosing to see our feelings in the light of love instead of fear, we take back our power. By surrendering control and embracing love we find healing. When you feel your feelings for 90 seconds, it allows a break-through to take place. It is scary, but you create space for peace by processing the hard feelings.

I am learning about Shamans and the work they do. Shamans believe that by naming diseases, you take them away, they have no power over you.[2] They view disease as an energetic imbalance. Finding balance in all things is key to our healing. By hiding in the darkness, you prolong your stay there.

You don't need to stay in the grey muddled mess permanently. You can choose growth, and your growth can be profound. Specific colors are meant to be seen and felt. In the next twenty-four hours, I want you to write down what you think is creating grey in your life. Be honest with yourself, because the more you resist, the more things persist! You are worthy of feeling peace and healing

---

[2] "5 Types of Imbalance: A Guide to Illness from a Shamanic Perspective." Sounds True

today, it doesn't have to take months. You can feel peace right now.

This book aims to help you understand that you are worthy of self-love. You deserve to finally see yourself through the Divine lens of infinite unconditional love. Don't give up because there is so much beauty to be seen. Together, we can discover the colors.

Chapter 4

The Mind Is A Garden

In December of 2022, I went on a family trip to Florida. I hadn't been to Florida before, so every experience was new. As luck would have it, I started my period halfway through our second week. When I start my period, my emotions seem heavier and more challenging to manage.

We had a beach day planned, and everything seemed to go wrong. We were late getting out the door. The kids kept bugging each other in the backseat. It was a long drive, we went to the wrong area, and to top it off, we couldn't even swim because the current was too strong. I was angry and overwhelmed, and the meticulously planned day seemed to fall apart. I wanted to go home.

My husband and I have this thing where we start days over. No matter what time during the day it is, we say, "Let's have a good day." We started doing this because I sometimes let small things ruin my day. A friend once asked me, "Did you have a bad day or a bad five minutes?" By her asking this simple but powerful question, I changed my perspective.

That is a lesson I have held onto for many years. Moments can be challenging, but that doesn't mean the entire day needs to be affected negatively. So, ask yourself, when you seem caught in a strong tide of it being a bad day, "Is it a bad day or a bad five minutes? Is it worth ruining my day over a bad five minutes?"

In a study led by the National Science Foundation, they say that our minds have an average of 12,000-60,000 thoughts a day, and that 80% of those thoughts are negative![3] The craziest part is that 95% are repeated thoughts from the previous days. Over and over, we allow negative thoughts to impact our lives. YOU have to change your thoughts and choose to have a good day, even if you had a bad five minutes.

You control the thoughts in your mind. When something happens, it may be painful at the time, but you allow the pain to continue by replaying it in your head repeatedly. That's why it is important to choose a good day consciously. We create unnecessary repeated pain by reliving an event in our minds. Choose to replace negativity with positivity. Reframe the negative five minutes you had and choose again.

---

[3] Verma, Prakhar. "Destroy Negativity from Your Mind with This Simple Exercise." Medium

So, in the moment at the beach, I decided to have a good day! I chose to change my mood. I reset my mood by taking the kids out and looking for seashells. It was beautiful; we could at least get our feet wet and find beautiful pieces of nature.

I like weird keepsake shit to remind me of lessons I have learned, and I wanted a seashell. I am picky about seashells, so I asked the Universe to help me find one. I needed a unique seashell. There had been rough moments throughout the day, and I wanted to know that the Universe was aware of me. After a few minutes of searching, I found one! It was pretty, but it wasn't the one I needed.

Discovering our motivation for our thoughts and actions is an essential tool in our healing journey. Another word for motivation is intention. What is your intention behind your existence? Is it love? As we make love the center of our existence, we create an environment of peace for others and ourselves. Establishing an intention of love allows you to start again. Release the negative emotions and move forward in a light of love regardless of the negativity you've experienced in a day.

> As we make love the center of our existence, we create an environment of peace for others and ourselves.

I genuinely desire everyone to feel the emotional freedom of loving ourselves fully. Because that is my desire, I check my intention behind my thoughts and actions. Am I helping this person because I genuinely just want to help? Am I doing it for ego-related reasons? Are my intentions that of love?

Be intentional in your thoughts and actions; by doing so, you will live more authentically surrounded by immense peace. Intention is powerful, learning what that means can truly be life changing. I highly recommend *The Power of Intention* by Wayne Dyer[4]. It truly changed my life and the way I connect with the Universe.

Our minds are like a garden. We need to be intentional about what we are planting in that garden. The more we care for specific thoughts, the more they grow. Our thoughts lead to actions. Are the plants we are growing worthy of our time and energy? Are we intentional about planting love, positivity, self-growth, etc., into our minds? Or do we allow judgment, self-criticism, and negativity to grow rapidly?

In his book, Wayne Dyer talks about the seven faces of intention, one of which is abundance. The Universe is infinitely abundant in all things. The Universe can provide whatever you seek: money, love, health, happiness, etc. We need to be willing and receptive, which receptivity is another one of Wayne's faces of intention.

When I wake up, I repeat, "I am love. I am kind. I am creative. I am beautiful. I am expansion. I am

---

[4] Dyer, Wayne W. *The power of intention*. Carlsbad, CA: Hay House, 2004.

abundance. I am receptivity." Those are all seven faces of intention.

From my experiences, I fully recognize that the Universe listens and is willing to provide when we ask using the power of intention. Focusing on love, kindness, creativity, beauty, expansion, abundance, and receptivity in all aspects of our lives is how we find answers from the Universe.

As I asked the Universe for a sign, I kept my intentional morning mantra in mind. I knew that the Universe is abundant and could provide me with a shell because the Universe is aware of me. It may seem silly to want a shell, but I needed to know that the Universe heard me and that I wasn't alone at that moment. I whispered, "Universe, I know you are abundant in all things and have infinite power. I am receptive and seeking a shell. Please, I know you can provide me with one that I need." After I whispered my little prayer, I got slammed with a wave that almost knocked me over! I was only at knee length, so it was a strong one!

On top of that, a shell hit me in the ankle. Not exactly the way I thought my answer would come, but my answer came. Sometimes we need to be smacked by the Universe to change our attitude and to help us recognize that "Hell yeah, Jamie, I am listening, and I always have your back!"

I asked for a sign, and the Universe provided one. I was willing and ready to receive. Are you? You may be praying or asking the Universe for things, but what are your intentions? Are your intentions aligned with the light of Divine power?

We must surrender our desired outcome to the goodness of the Universe; and trust that Divine understanding is a journey, not a destination. Aligning our desires with the Universe is how we do things through the power of intention. The Universe will provide Divine understanding as we seek genuine understanding in all things.

I struggle with seeing myself as beautiful. When I get upset because my pants don't fit right or my face looks rounder, what are my intentions behind those thoughts? Are they thoughts created out of love, or thoughts created out of judgment? As I shift my focus to the reasoning and intention that created those thoughts, I am able to see truths and false beliefs. I no longer focus on the minuscule negative thoughts that take place, because I intentionally love myself. I choose every day to see beauty. My pant size doesn't matter, but the amount of love I hold for myself does.

The Universe is full of intentional love, so take time to connect to that. Sit and meditate on your personal intentions behind your thoughts and the way you are living your life. What are your intentions in what you seek? Are you willing to follow through with the guidance the Universe gives? Do you BELIEVE the Universe is abundant in all things? Believing that the Universe has limitations holds us back from the greatness we are meant to achieve.

Regardless of our emotional state, we can always turn to the Universe. It is full of infinite love and understanding. If a slam to the ankle wasn't a big enough sign, the Universe gave me another sign to make me aware of Universe's infinite abundance in all things.

After our time at the beach, we had a guided kayaking tour. We were going through Mangrove trees, where Manatees frequently reside. The idea of seeing a freaking manatee in real life had me stoked!

My husband and the guide saw a baby, but I wasn't close enough. I put my hands on the water and surrendered my desire to the Universe with a prayer. In prayer, I told the Universe I knew its infinite power and that nothing is impossible. I asked to see a manatee.

We continued our trip, and I kept an eye out for manatees, but I didn't spot any. Our tour was almost over, and I had given up on seeing a manatee. I was disappointed, but I thanked the Universe for our beautiful adventure. It was genuinely magical kayaking through the Mangrove trees with my little family. The sun was setting, and we witnessed an exquisite sunset.

As we watched the sunset, we saw a dolphin on our last stretch back to where we had started! The dolphin jumped out of the water and was magnificent. It continued jumping out of the water while escorting us back to our starting point. The magnificence of that creature was fucking spectacular, along with the perfect timing!

When I was younger, I wanted to be a marine mammal trainer and work with dolphins. Then as

I got a little older, I wanted to be a marine biologist but was still obsessed with dolphins.

So, seeing one in the wild was truly magical. I knew that the Universe truly was listening. I received an answer, and though it wasn't the one I thought it would be, it was beautiful.

That is the crazy thing about the power of the Universe. We sometimes receive answers in the most unexpected ways. I didn't know I would see a dolphin while kayaking through an orange sunset on the spectacular waters of Florida. I was hoping for a manatee, but what I received was much more beautiful than I initially hoped.

As we keep ourselves in a receptive mindset, the answers we receive will be the ones that are of our highest good. Wayne Dyer gave a powerful meditation statement: "I accept the guidance and assistance of the same force that created me, I let go of my ego, and I trust in this wisdom to move at its own peaceful pace. I make no demands on it." When I asked to see a manatee, I knew the Universe was in control. I didn't demand, I surrendered my desire to the Universe. I trusted that whatever happened was meant to be.

As I traveled in peace, I kept my eyes open to the possibility of seeing a manatee, but I didn't force it. I didn't jump in the water, desperately seeking one out. I allowed the answers to come their way and in their own time.

Gabby Bernstein talks a lot about stepping out of the way of the Universe and trusting that answers will come. I did a 21-day manifesting challenge with Gabby. She tells you to pick a sign from the Universe to let you know if you are heading in the right direction and then surrender to the outcome. A sign can be anything of significance to you. Just a reminder that you aren't alone, and that hope still exists in the darkness.

For example, I love Sunflowers. When I am struggling, Sunflowers seem to pop up more, as a reminder that I am not alone in the Universe. There are also number signs, this is called numerology. Numerology[5] is believing in a mystical or divine relationship between numbers and coinciding events. There is a term within numerology called angel numbers[6]. These numbers are sequences of usually three and four numbers that contain repetition.

I have been seeing 111 a lot, which can mean a lot of things. But to me, it means I am being guided by my Divine Guardians, letting me know I am on the path I am meant to be on. It doesn't matter how alone you feel; the Universe is aware of you.

Gabby says to forget about your chosen sign and go about your day. You can't force a sign from the Universe. The Universe will show up and give you your sign, but not receiving a sign can also be a sign! It is all about surrendering your will and ego to the Universe! Trust the process, and

---

[5] Decoz, Hans. "What Is Numerology?" What is Numerology | World Numerology, 2022.

[6] Staff, Numerology. "Your Guide to Angel Number Meanings." Numerology.com, 2023.

know that you deserve to see yourself through the Divine lens of unconditional and infinite love that the Universe offers.

I asked the Universe for specific signs with the seashell and the manatee. I trusted in the ultimate abundant power of the Universe. I released my ego and accepted that the Universe wants my best and highest self. As I align myself with the love of the Universe, I will see the power it offers to work through me to achieve the greatest good for myself and those around me. I deserve to see myself through infinite and unconditional love.

It doesn't matter what "flaws" you have. You are worthy of loving yourself unconditionally. What does unconditional love look like? I am still learning. Unconditional love means you won't give up on yourself. You take your spiritual growth and healing seriously. Loving yourself isn't something that just happens, it takes work. It takes reframing your negative thoughts, and looking for signs from the Universe.

Loving yourself means you give yourself kindness, you look for times to feel love from the Universe. There is an infinite amount of love that surrounds you. The Universe is willing and ready to provide signs to show you an abundance of love. All you have to do is ask!

The Universe surrounds us with infinite love that wants us to succeed. We will live on a higher vibration as we release the need to control the outcome and trust that the Universe has our back. We will be able to lift others and empower them to reside on the highest vibration of love.

Step into your power, and know that as you surrender to the will of the Universe, you will experience daily enlightenment. The Universe will guide you toward the answers you are seeking because the Universe is aware of you. Choose today to be receptive and open to answers. Have an open heart and allow the guidance to flow through you. You, my dear, are worth all the positive, energetic power the Universe offers.

Take ten minutes today, and sit in meditation. What is it that you are truly seeking in your life right now? Every day I seek to be surrounded by love and light. I don't want to live in my darkness anymore. I choose to trust the Universe that each day holds light for me. As you seek, answers will come. Don't try to force them. Just listen. Put your hands on the water and surrender your desire to the Universe.

Chapter 5

The Power of Pause

At the beginning of 2022, I completed an apprenticeship/schooling to become a dog groomer! Let me tell you, friend -- I had yet to learn how difficult dog grooming was. It is like cutting a human's hair, except the human moves, bites, licks, and doesn't listen. I learned many different tricks, tools, and skills during this schooling.

When grooming dogs, you use skills from reading their energy to knowing what direction to hold your scissors. There is a reason groomers put in a significant amount of time getting trained!

One of the main lessons I learned during this apprenticeship was that grooming is a skill that needs to be taught, practiced, and practiced some more. Well, I now groom from home and have seen some crazy stuff. A few days ago, I had a woman reach out to me who had been struggling to get into groomers because they were all booked. This woman attempted to groom her dog from home.

She sent me a picture of her dog, and damn, it was rough.

That poor dog looked like it got run over by a lawn mower, and to top it off, it was a poodle. In my opinion, poodles are the most brutal damn dogs to groom. The need for professional skills is apparent if you aren't trained and try to groom your dog from home.

There is a reason everyone has different skill sets, and relying on others' skills doesn't make us weak. It takes great strength to ask for help in areas we lack.

I groomed her poodle. It was a lot of work, but we got it looking how she wanted! Her grooming made it harder for me to groom the dog, because I had to work around her haircut. I couldn't go with my typical grooming lines or scissor how I normally would. It would have been easier to have her bring me her dog originally, because I would've spent less time fixing the cut.

But because of pride, a lack of resources, etc. we don't always ask for help right away. We can't do everything, and by trying to do it all we will burn ourselves out.

The woman with the poodle didn't have the expertise to groom her dog, and it showed. But she did reach out to someone who did. I got her dog scheduled, and we were able to do a beautiful haircut. Sometimes we must call on others' skills and expertise to help us.

My dad was a single parent for most of my childhood, so he was forced to do everything for me and my two older sisters. My mom passed away when I was two, which meant my dad took over hair duty. My dad became Mr. Mom to three girls under the age of eight. He did his best with my hair, but girls' hair was outside his skill set.

My dad admitted to using a potato chip clip for a hairpiece once, so though my hair looked like a complete disaster, my dad had the best intentions when attempting hairstyles. It was just out of his scope of skills. So, it helped when my oldest sister, Allie, learned how to do hair. We were all grateful because parenting three girls is hard enough without worrying about crazy hair.

If someone's strength differs from your own, it is okay to ask for help. Whether it is dog grooming, learning how to do hair, or reading a book about learning various mindfulness meditation skills, relying on others' skills takes humility. We can't do everything, and that is okay.

A friend recently asked me what my favorite coping skill is when struggling. I responded that I have been learning the art of not responding immediately. Suppose I feel triggered by my kid or husband, then I need to take a minute and breathe. I then ask myself if my reaction will hurt them, and if it will, is that hurt I will cause worth my reaction? The answer is no, and the hurt anger causes is not worth that reaction.

My anger or reaction isn't worth the hurt it would cause those I love. So, I breathe. I have started doing what I call my mediation minute. The amount of time spent meditating doesn't matter. What matters is the intention you have when practicing a meditation minute. During my meditation minute, I focus on what matters: love. Is what I am doing or saying going to help those around me feel loved? If it isn't, then it isn't worth my energy. On your healing journey, during your meditation minutes, put energy into love and authenticity. Anything beyond that is just an exhausting waste of energy. Learning skills takes time, but the more you heal yourself, the easier it is for you to be a source of love to those around you.

Learning new parenting skills has become essential to my growth as a human. Parenting isn't easy, and the longer I am a mom, the more I learn the importance of taking a breath. Breathing is a learned practiced skill, and I didn't realize how hard it is until I became a mom!

My 2-year-old daughter, Kambria, has started this new thing where she grabs onto her 4-year-old brother's hair and just yanks. She will have both hands gripped like she is about to fall off a ledge into a pool of alligators. She is relentless. It has been challenging because we are trying to teach her healthy ways to express her feelings besides hurting her brother.

Well, one day, I was fed up. They had constantly been fighting, and my patience was low. She grabbed a couple of handfuls of Ryker's hair and pulled. I smacked her hand to get her to let it go. I could have opened her fingers, pulled him away, or done many other things. But I chose to smack her hand. She let go and ran into the other room to her dad, crying.

My heart just broke. I knew that was not the way to handle her big emotions. My son was crying, she was crying, and now I was crying because I felt like the world's shittiest mom. I had to look inward and figure out why I was so angry. Why did I allow the actions of a 2-year-old to trigger emotions intense enough that I smacked her hand? Since they were old enough to hit, I have told my children that hands should be used to uplift, love, and strengthen others, not hurt people.

My husband came and got Ryker so I could have a moment, and they went and watched a movie in the living room. I did a meditative prayer and asked the Universe to help me change. It is all about practicing our new skills, and breathing is a skill I need to practice more!

The coping skill I used when my husband gave me space was my tapping breathing. It is where you tap various parts of your body while taking deep centered breaths, and repeating various affirmations or sayings. I also reflected on where my anger was coming from. By finding the source of that frustration, I was able to acknowledge it, and move past it.

A spilled cup of chocolate milk is not worth your inner peace! Accidents happen, mistakes transpire, but nothing is worth your inner peace. I am not perfect at this, but I am trying.

After I took my mediation minute, I went to where my family was watching the movie and asked Kambria if we could talk. That sweet girl said yes, and we walked hand in hand to her bedroom. I knelt to her level and explained that sometimes Mommy has big feelings and doesn't express them how she should, but that I was learning. I told her that using my hands to hurt her wasn't acceptable and that I should never use my hands to hurt others. I explained that our hand's purpose is to help, love, and heal and that I was wrong for how I responded. I also explained that pulling hair isn't something we do either and explained the same concept of using kind hands.

That conversation with my daughter was one of the most powerful teaching moments I have ever experienced. It taught me that life isn't about ego, and it isn't about being right. Life is about doing what is right, and my choice to hit my daughter's hand was wrong. Although she is two and probably won't remember that conversation, I hope that opens a door for us to talk about big feelings and feel safe about owning our mistakes. Life is all about learning skills and having experiences that teach us growth.

I was talking to my therapist about feeling like a shitty mom. She said my guilt isn't helping them or me, it is creating a negative energy of judgement. I am not a perfect mom, but by taking time to talk to my kid when I fuck up allows an understanding and learning of growth. My kids won't be perfect, but by having the conversations after mistakes are made, it will teach them to embrace growth. We can't throw imperfections in our faces, but we can continuously choose to turn to love instead of judgement. We can't guilt ourselves into change, we can only love ourselves into change.

To grow spiritually, we must learn tools that guide us through our healing. Steps that may seem minor right now, could make the world of difference tomorrow. Don't hold the mistakes of the past, or who you used to be over your head anymore. Recognize that change is part of life, and life is just an opportunity to experience growth. Guilt doesn't serve you, it just fucks up your energy of peace and growth.

Changing a little each day isn't easy. Recognizing things we can change, and then learning the tools to do so, takes time. The fuller our tool belt is, the easier it will be to manage strong emotions that create negativity. Living with a larger perspective means expanding your toolbelt of skills so you can take time to see the bigger picture.

Another tool we have been implementing when we are upset is blowing out candles. Figuratively blowing out candles helps if you have littles, but I do it when alone too. You hold up your hand and blow out the number of candles on your hand. This exercise allows you to redirect your mind to something silly and always focus on your breathing.

It is okay not to be a perfect mom, friend, daughter, brother, etc. Our purpose isn't to be perfect, our purpose is to grow. Every day we can change a little, learn tools to be better and share divine love even when we have big feelings.

The Universe is in constant care of you, and as you take time to do meditation minutes, the Universe will guide you in the direction of growth. We can change day by day, minute by minute. I don't need to be the angry mom who smacks her kid's hand because I choose to change. I choose to take my time and remember that no negative emotion is worth my peace and the peace of those I love.

Choosing to change takes time, and meditation minutes take practice. There is a powerful meditative practice called the power of pause. The world is in a constant state of chaos and isn't showing signs of quieting down.

Chaos breeds chaos. That is why the power of pause is essential. Our souls crave quiet and silence because that is when we grow and connect to our Divine. The chaos can become overwhelming if we aren't taking those moments to connect to the Universe. We need tranquility to breed peace instead of allowing chaos to breed chaos. The power of pause is a process that can create healing in our souls.

Growth is a process, but as I pause and reflect on what matters, that is when I become a better wife, mom, friend, etc., I change simply by sitting in the silence. So often, we respond immediately, and it makes things worse. Learning the Power of Pause is a skill that requires practice and patience.

We need tranquility to breed peace instead of allowing chaos to breed chaos.

Like any skill, the Power of Pause is a learned skill. Creating inner silence is necessary to help you navigate Divine enlightenment. When I need a quick meditation minute to practice the power of pause, I focus on breathing. I go into a quiet corner of my house and take five breaths in, hold it for five seconds, then exhale for five seconds. I do this over and over. As I focus on this simple breathing technique, I create inner peace. I quiet my mind and the noise around me to connect to what matters most, love.

When I was twelve years old, I got a dog named Lizzie. She was there for me through my dad and stepmom's divorce and my early adulthood. She was my girl.

When I was twenty-two, I had to put her down. That was one of the most challenging experiences I have ever gone through. We had an appointment to put Lizzie down. The night before she died, I took her to the kitchen and sat on the floor with her. That night I sang to her, held her, and cried. I said goodbye to my best friend. I decided that night to make clay imprints of her feet.

Seven years later, I carried that imprinted clay piece with me as we moved through five different houses. We were packing to move again, and somehow my kids got ahold of the clay piece. I am unsure of how or where they even found it. But they did. When a four-year-old and a three-year-old get ahold of something valuable, it inevitably winds up broken. And that is precisely what happened.

I immediately yelled and cried when I saw that they had broken it. My son yelled when I yelled because he didn't know why mom was so upset. They were simply playing. When he yelled and started crying, I immediately shifted my focus to him. Lizzie is a dog I will remember for the rest of my life. It broke my heart when my kids broke the clay, but seeing that my reaction hurt my son impacted me even more.

The clay breaking was devastating, but only for a moment. Seeing that I hurt Ryker brought me out of my grief. I knew that at the moment, Ryker was what mattered. Those around us are what matter. That isn't to say my feelings were invalid, but is it worth hurting those we love?

The clay piece is fixable. Though it won't be the same, it is still fixable. But our words and reactions to those around us aren't always fixable. Our meditation minutes are essential because they allow us to see the bigger picture. The words I say during those moments of devastation, exhaustion, or darkness can impact my son for years.

My older sister, Jackie, is one of the best humans I have ever met. The kindness that radiates from her is perceivable to every person she meets. The older I get, the more I realize that my sister is one of a kind. She is simply the best.

I have learned from her the impact of words. Words aren't easily forgotten and can create lasting damage. If she gets in a fight with anyone, she just shuts the hell up. She doesn't say unkind words, even if she knows what would stab you the deepest. She just shuts up.

Sticks and stones may break bones, but words will cause damage, requiring therapy and long-term healing. So, when my son broke that piece of clay, and I saw that my anger was affecting him, it immediately allowed me to flip my switch. I took deep breaths and realized nothing was worth hurting my sweet little boy.

No sadness that we feel, no anger that arises, and no frustration that exhumes from us is worth hurting those we love. That is not to say those feelings are invalid or shouldn't be expressed, but if they hurt another, they must be released differently.

That is why having an imaginary tool belt with various coping mechanisms is essential. According to Albert Einstein, the definition of insanity is trying the same thing over and over and expecting different results.

If you don't build your toolbelt, how can you expect to react differently in triggering or challenging situations? Various coping mechanisms allow us to respond in a way that helps us feel those feelings but still permits awareness and validation.

There is a saying I frequently use for myself and my kiddos. When we need to breathe, I ask if we need some "calm downtown time." Calm downtown time can be sitting in our room for a few minutes by ourselves, cuddling on the couch, taking deep breaths to blow out the figurative candles on our hands, or whatever healthy coping mechanisms we want to use.

When I recognized that I was triggered by Ryker breaking the piece of clay, I had to ask for calm downtown time. I want my kids to fill their emotional tool belts by showing them that validating our feelings is okay and there are healthy ways to express them. I can teach them there is safety in feelings and freedom when we don't suppress feelings.

Rewiring our brains is challenging and takes daily practice. But continuously trying to do things that bring light and love into our lives is how we begin to change. The clay mold is something I can fix, and how I speak and react to my children is something I can control. We must decide to change, react differently, and be a beacon of light and positivity.

So, friend, I hope you are kind to yourself and remember that perfection isn't necessary, but growth is. Ego isn't necessary, but love is. You are worth the energy it takes to learn the meditative power of pause skill and the time to experience mediation minutes. Like grooming a dog, navigating our emotions and pausing is a learned skill. Be kind to yourself as you learn, remember you can't guilt yourself into change. You can only love yourself into change.

Your divine Spirit will step into the connection and power of the Universe each time you take a minute to pause and breathe. You are worthy of Divine self-love regardless of how often you react instead of breathing. Seeing yourself through an unconditional, infinite Divine love is possible. Take the time to learn meditation minutes and the power of pause because you deserve to see yourself through the Divine lens of infinite unconditional love.

Before reading more, take a minute to pause and write some of the coping mechanisms you can use next time you feel triggered. Having coping mechanisms you've prepped in advance will help you from scrambling the next time you feel triggered. In the moment it can seem overwhelming to switch our frame of mind. Three things. You can do it; write three things to help you next time you feel triggered! Remember, healing is found when we take baby steps forward.

Chapter 6

Reason, Season, or For Life!

Recently, I had a dear friendship end. Without warning or a real reason, she ghosted me. She truly didn't give me a reason until a couple of months later, but even then, her reasoning didn't make sense, and we didn't talk in person. I learned from that experience what people think of us is truly none of our business. She had her issues and her perspective. Her ending the relationship was solely a her thing.

Sometimes people just don't want us in their lives, and that is okay; the people worth our energy will reciprocate our energy. Friendship break-ups are real though, and they are truly devastating. I have had a few friendship break-ups, and each one taught me to love myself a little more instead of relying on others' love to fulfill me.

Her friendship was one that I thought would be a lifelong friendship and one that taught me so many things. But I learned more from that relationship ending than I ever did during it. There is a power in becoming our own best friend, and I hope this book helps you embrace that power. The relationships we have are ever-evolving. I learned that people come into our lives for a reason, a season, or for life.

I was talking to one of my best friends about this relationship ending. I told her I felt broken and surrounded by so much pain. She told me something I will never forget and strive to live up to every day. She said, "Jamie, you are an honor to know. Whether knowing you briefly on a beach or building an intimate lifelong relationship with you, it is an honor. If people don't recognize that, then bye!"

Hearing those words from someone I love and trust significantly lifted my heart and helped me recognize my worth. I am worthy of divine friendships that lift and strengthen me. We all are. Every day the people you surround yourself with influence your life. Are they lifting us to a higher vibration or bringing us down?

We all live on different vibrations. At Estuary, I learned about something called 11+. Before I went to Estuary, I lived daily at vibrations 1-10. One feeling not so great, having a dark day, and ten feeling amazing. Each day we can find ourselves on various numbers within the scale. But we can live beyond that scale.

As we connect to our higher power and live on a vibration of positivity and love, we can live at 11+. Our "hard days" don't have to fall below 11 because we feel our great divinity. Each day as we spend time connecting to the Universe, we are placing ourselves on a higher frequency of living.

You may seek validation outside of yourself or others' acceptance, approval, and recognition. As you turn to sources outside of yourself, you automatically lower your vibration of living. Deep within yourself is a supreme spirit, which is your true identity! Your true identity is full of peace and all-knowing!

Your dark days don't have to be pitch black. You can release the emptiness of that darkness because you no longer live on a scale of 1-10. You can trust that the Universe is genuinely guiding you to live on the frequency of 11+.

Each day as we spend time connecting to the Universe, we are placing ourselves on a higher frequency of living.

I appreciated that one of my best friends told me I am an honor to know. I am now at a place where I say that to myself and believe it. To live at 11+, filling our cup is a necessity. I can't rely on others to pull me out of the darkness or tell me affirmations I should be telling myself.

What are the reasons we aren't living at 11+? Is it mental health? Triggers? Self-talk? We aren't living on our highest vibration for a million reasons, so let's talk about some of those reasons.

Let's talk triggers. When I was hospitalized for my first suicide attempt, there was one lesson I learned that changed my view on depression. Depression is like a pot of water on the stove; it gets bubblier and bubblier until it starts to go over.

I recognize when my depression is starting to appear. My self-talk becomes more negative, I snap easier at dumb shit, just little signs here and there. Looking inward, I know when that darkness starts to bubble in my soul.

How are you speaking to yourself every day? Living on a higher vibration means we are intentional about the thoughts in our heads. If we are speaking to ourselves negatively every day, we can't truly be living on a frequency of 11+.

Is a chemical imbalance keeping you from living 11+? There is a gross stigmatization of medicine. I was ashamed that I needed medicine to balance me. I got medicinal help when I needed it. There is nothing wrong with turning to a doctor for help. I no longer use medications, but there was a time when my medication is what kept my head above water. There is no shame in that, so if a chemical imbalance is what is keeping you from 11+, why not get the help you need?

Another reason I find myself living on lower vibrations are when I am lacking in my commitment to meditation, or not finding quiet time for myself each day. Finding time to hang out with me allows me to fill my cup from within without needing others approval or acceptance. As I focus on the quiet moments with myself I block out the negativity of others and live on a higher vibration.

Have you heard of shadow work? Shadow work is when we face the feelings we are experiencing instead of suppressing them.[7] Shadowwork is a healing modality for the brave who want to face repressed pieces of themselves that have been buried. Positive aspects are in the shadow, so through shadow work our goal is to discover what those are.

Shadow work is us processing our triggers, not suppressing them. Doing so strengthens our Spirit, allowing us to handle outside situations easier. It is the sweetest healing version because it reveals your golden shadow, which is your true self. Shadow work is not a one and done healing activity. It is a process, and doing it frequently allows true healing.

In essence, it means going into your darkness. What are you avoiding, and do you have the courage to look it in the face and battle your demons?

For years, I have seen my depression as a giant green monster. She sits in the room with me, sometimes on my lap, overwhelming my space or just peeking through the door at a distance. But I

---

[7] Fosu, Kimberly. "Shadow Work: A Simple Guide to Transcending the Darker Aspects of the Self." Medium.

have seen that monster and have allowed her in my space.

When I feel my green depression monster trying to step in, there is a specific meditation I have started doing. This form of shadow work helps me understand the triggers behind my depression.

This specific shadow work meditation is me visualizing myself in my home, and when "depression" decides to knock on my door, I open the door and acknowledge the presence of depression. I say hello, and figure out why she is visiting. I validated her feelings and the reasons behind her visit.

So how do you figure out why a specific emotion came up? You sit in it, and allow whatever thoughts enter your mind to flow through. There is something called the emotional wheel. A quick google search will show you that there are emotions beyond the primary ones we feel. So by validating the reasoning behind a depressive visit, I can further understand the deeper emotions I am feeling.

My depression would visit a lot because I had genuine feelings of disdain towards myself. It's scary to feel that darkness, but feeling it allows me to get to the root of the problem. Understand that by addressing the darkness, you can take away the fear. By removing the fear, you discover the reason behind the visit from your emotions. As you release fear, your perspective shifts to a lens of love.

We must look the darkness in the eye and allow those suppressed feelings to be felt. It can be so hard to feel those feelings. I would know, I love to avoid feelings. I am a professional suppressor. But suppressing feelings denies growth.

I close my meditation when I have fully addressed various triggers and understand why she is there. I close by thanking her for coming, wishing her well, and sending her on her way. Having an attitude of gratitude raises vibrations, which is why I always thank my feelings for coming up.

I no longer allow depression to come in uninvited, overwhelm my space, and take up unwanted time. By validating my depression, I don't suppress my feelings. Feelings or triggers always come up for a reason, and as we acknowledge them, we allow emotional processing to begin and gain a greater understanding of the world around us. We allow healing to be our guide instead of being driven by fear those feelings can create.

My giant green depressive monster no longer controls me, and I choose every day to live on a higher vibration of 11+. My "dark days" are not that dark because I can no longer sink to 1-10. My "most amazing days" of living at a ten were barely scraping the surface of divine happiness.

There is so much goodness the Universe has to offer us. It is not always easy to live at 11+, but as we choose daily to connect to the higher source of the Universe, we can live on this higher vibration. Plant new seeds within yourself. Now is the time to eliminate lower vibrational living and adopt new and higher vibrational habits.

As you replenish yourself, you naturally replenish your connection to the higher power of the Universe. Cultivate the strength and sense of your existence! The magical connection to the Divine will enhance your spiritual and material resources.

You no longer need to live in a desperate vibration, begging for things. You can trust that the Universe provides and desires your happiness. Every day is a chance for a new beginning.

When I make a mistake, I say to myself, "In the same moment." I say this because I can choose to change at the exact moment. I can choose to be better and learn every day. Every day we have the opportunity to change, and a day when we don't change just a little is a missed opportunity!

I deserve to see myself through the Divine lens of infinite, unconditional love! No mistake has made me beyond the reach of that Divine self-love, and every day I can feel that infinite love.

Growth is necessary, and we can experience it daily. Even taking an extra minute to breathe and thank the Universe for the tremendous power you hold within can be enough growth for a day.

You are an honor to know, and every day as you strive to live on your highest vibration, the people you rub shoulders with will feel that light you bring to every interaction, even if it is a simple 10-minute conversation with a stranger. You are an honor to know. Regardless of the reason, season, or lifelong interactions you have, your presence is an honor.

I challenge you to use this affirmation as you look in the mirror today. "I am an honor to know and every person with whom I interact is for a reason, season, or life. I am an honor to know. I live at 11+ because I connect daily to my Divine power. I find peace within myself and no longer seek love or validation from outside sources. I am enough as I am; the Universe infinitely loves me."

You will not succumb to the darkness if you validate it. I promise. Your light is stronger than the darkness you feel. You are not alone, you are not a burden, and you, my dear, are an honor to know.

Chapter 7

You Choose The Relationships You Attract

In January 2022, we took a weekend and celebrated my birthday. On this weekend, I had two of the scariest experiences I have ever had in my life. My husband and I decided to take our kiddos to the hot springs, an hour-and-a-half drive away. We are in Wyoming, and January can get a shit ton of snow! But today, the sun was shining, so we drove through the canyon to the springs.

As we were driving, I lost control of the car, which spun out. We landed in a three-foot snow bank and were stuck. The terror that filled my body was immediate. I had my entire family in the car. Their lives were in my hands, and I lost control. I was engulfed in the fear of losing them. The terror of the car spinning out with our screams is engraved into my brain.

I will thank the Universe that we were all okay for the rest of our lives. Our car was stuck, and there wasn't a thing we could do about it ourselves. Fortunately, a cute older couple stopped and started helping us dig with our dinky window scraper.

We tried pushing it out, and it just got us more stuck. Well, another car stopped, and this car had a mom and two sons. Together we kept digging! Thankfully, a snow plow came, and he had a shovel in his truck. He allowed us to borrow his shovel and said to stick it in the snow when we finished, and he would grab it on his way back.

The shovel made a difference, but we still couldn't get out. Another car stopped, and that car had a family of four. All of us took turns digging, and we pushed again. No luck. After this second push, I was in the driver's seat and whispered a prayer to the Universe. I said, "Dear Universe, I am grateful that we are all safe and that all these people have stopped to help us get out. We have done all we can but need your help to get out. Please, help us get out of this."

I opened my eyes and started to get out of my car. Before I even opened my door, a blue truck pulled up, and this was the answer to my little prayer. This truck had tow straps, quickly hooked us up, and gave us a yank! Within minutes we were out of the snow and back on the road. The gratitude I felt to the Universe for that IMMEDIATE answer was overwhelming. As we drove, my family and I said a thank you prayer to the Universe.

So many people showed up, and over ten stopped to help us. No one needed to stop, but people are inherently good.

In high school, I wore a necklace that said, "Be the change you wish to see in the world." Every day I strive to live by that, but that day I saw that quote through random strangers who helped a family in need.

We had a couple of cars pass us instead of helping, and a part of my ego wanted to pass judgment. They were trucks, and I wondered why they wouldn't stop to help. But then I realized I couldn't pass judgment because I didn't know their situation. An important lesson popped into my head after this happened: if you can show someone kindness, do it! But don't pass judgment on those who don't have the space to be present.

So often, we get caught up in thinking that someone else will do it, or wondering what they may think of you. More often than not, people will be grateful and appreciate kindness versus thinking other thoughts. We need more kindness in the world, and it starts from within.

People showed another act of kindness to me at the pool when my second scariest moment happened. My husband took our son to the bathroom, and I was sitting with my feet in the hot tub watching our daughter, with her swim vest, play in the kiddy pool. I looked away for less than 10 seconds, but when I looked back, I saw my sweet, two-year-old babe face down in the pool. I ran and got her out as quickly as I could. She was in ten inches of water. Ten inches deep, and I almost lost her. Had I not been watching, I very well could have.

To see your child not struggling or even moving with their face in the water is a haunting picture. I remember yelling and sprinting into the water as quickly as possible. I picked up her little body, hoping that no damage was done. She was coughing and crying, I was crying, and we just held each other.

I will thank the Universe every day that I didn't lose her. Seeing her like that was extremely traumatizing, and my mama heart is still recovering. She is fine, and was more upset that I was holding her outside the pool instead of letting her continue to play! But as I was holding her, another mom came over and said, "You did good, mama. You were fast. Is there anything I can do to help her?" I just looked at this woman, shrugged, cried, and held my daughter. I think I was in a bit of shock.

I took a minute to calm down, and my husband was back by then. My daughter went back to the pool with my husband, and I took some time to do a meditation minute. I needed to connect to the Universe because my heart was full of fear, and I wanted to transform it into gratitude.

When I stood up, I looked for that mom, we spotted each other across the pool, and I just whispered *thank you*. Her words of kindness and willingness to help were such a blessing. Though I didn't know how to respond when the accident happened, my heart was whole because she was there. She didn't know me, but she was immediately checking to see if she could help.

Both of these experiences were extremely dark and scary for me. But they taught me that I am not alone. People came to my rescue and showed me kindness because they saw someone in need and wanted to help. Isn't that all we can do as a society? Reach out to those in need. We can't always help, but showing up and creating space for others is sometimes all the help people need. You are NOT a burden; people will show up simply because there are good people.

Sometimes I feel alone, but as I meditate, I invite various energies to join me and fill me with their wisdom and love. During a specific meditation, I imagine myself at a conference table. This conference table has specific energies of people I have invited into my space. Each energy I have invited gives me further guidance for various questions or topics.

I do this meditation a lot with my mom. Doing this meditation has helped me receive guidance and feel comforted in times of need from her. My mom passed away from Lupus when I was two-years-old. So, finding different ways to fill that void of being motherless has become an essential part of my healing.

My conference table meditation has taught me that people's love and help go beyond this physical world. Albert Einstein said it best by saying, "Energy cannot be created or destroyed, it can only be changed from one form to another." By allowing various energies to give guidance and love, I grow my spiritual understanding of the people and energies in the Universe.

I expand my perspective on the way I see things. This meditation continuously teaches me that everyone is extraordinary. Treating other people like they are extraordinary will attract energies that live on a higher vibration. Whether physically or spiritually.

The Universe has our best intentions in mind, and the power of love surrounds us always. All we have to do is tune in. This meditation has become so powerful to me because I take time to listen to the Universe.

In *The Power of Intention*, Wayne Dyer says meditation is a time to listen to God speak. Regardless of what you call your Divine, the concept is the same. I know there is something greater than me that provides infinite amounts of love.

We are not alone; though we may feel like it sometimes. There are good and kind people willing to give love. If you are lonely, ask the Universe to send you a sign of comfort. Whether you meditate and create your spiritual conference table or choose another form of meditation, the Universe will show you your sign.

If you are open to receiving it, the Universe always provides. We have to choose to step into the abundant view of receiving. Manifesting healthy friendships around you will bring a sense of community into your life. If you live on high vibrational levels, you will receive what you put out there: strangers, angelic energies, or physical friendships will flock to that same high vibration. The same is true to lower vibrational living. You attract what you put out there.

If you seek healthy, like-minded friendships, that is what you will find. You will grow toxic relationships if you desperately seek others because you believe they will fill your cup. That is how the power of attraction works. Even if you don't believe in it, you automatically radiate energy. The type of energy you radiate is up to you.

It is time to release what doesn't serve your highest good and embrace the abundance of love the Universe offers.

High-energy people and high-energy angels surround us. It is all about our intention. Here is an affirmation I want you to add to your tool belt. Grab a sticky note, and put this on your mirror or somewhere you will see it daily! "I create healthy relationships in my life. I am worthy of surrounding myself with the highest vibration the Universe offers. I choose to see good in others and to be a source of peace, hope, and safety. I am enough and invite goodness and love into my inner circle."

Whether it is strangers on the street or angels on your pillow, you are worthy of healthy, loving relationships. It takes strength to see what doesn't serve your highest good. It is time to release what doesn't serve your highest good and embrace the abundance of love the Universe offers.

Chapter 8

Look In The Mirror

Every morning when I get my 2-year-old daughter from her room, we stop in front of her mirror. Together we repeat positive affirmations. "I am strong. I am beautiful. I am loved. I am worthy of love. I am healthy. I love my body. I am happy. I am smart." On and on and on. After that, we go on with our day.

As an adult, I realize the importance of shifting my focus inward to find truth in my affirmations. I want to help her find the truth in affirmations sooner than I did!

Recently, my family and I were touring new homes for a move. One of the houses we toured was staged beautifully with a 4-foot mirror. Ryker and Kambria immediately ran to that mirror and looked at each other. Ryker put his arm around Kambria and started saying positive affirmations.

I almost started crying as I watched them do this small activity together. I realized that Ryker caught on to my daily activity with Kambria. The way we speak to ourselves and those around us matters. Children notice, so we must ensure that self-positivity and love are what we are radiating. Ryker and I do affirmations occasionally when we catch ourselves in front of a mirror, but I was surprised at how aware he was.

Together, these sweet siblings repeated words I hope they remember for the rest of their lives. As we spend time lifting ourselves, we can lift others. As we build and establish self-love, we can look at those around us and help them see what we see.

They are building habits to see themselves through the Divine lens of infinite, unconditional love. Unconditional love is a learned skill because, for some reason, we allow the world to impact how we view ourselves. We must learn to shift our focus inward and allow the Universe to show us the love we hold. We are infinite beings, created from a Source so abundant in love. As we consistently say affirmations, we will eventually see ourselves through the lens of unconditional love. It takes time, but you are worth the time healing takes.

At Christmas, my children received a Moonlite phone projector. It is a cute little projector that uses your flashlight and an app to project stories onto the ceiling. Reading to my children at night is one of my favorite activities, so having a cool new twist on reading excited me!

We tried out the projector, and it didn't work. It was so freaking blurry, and I got so annoyed every time! The projector book was something I specifically requested in our group family Christmas chat. My hopes were high, and I was disappointed and frustrated. I tried for about a week with the little projector, but finally, my frustrations got the best of me, and I quit.

We were shopping around Walmart, and I saw a Walmart version of the little projector! It just came with a book and was like a mini projector flashlight. I tried it, and guess what? It was freaking blurry!

At this point, I was highly annoyed. I only wanted to spend some time doing something unique with my kids!

I gave the projector to my husband, who couldn't fix it either. It was only visible when it was about five inches from the wall. My husband said that was the distance it had to be, which didn't make sense. There had to be a different solution.

I was messing around with the Walmart one and almost dropped it, but I ended up twisting the front piece. Until now, I had yet to learn there was a front piece that twisted! As I twisted it, I realized the knob is how you focus the picture and eliminate the blur!

After all this freaking time and me walking away from a toy frustrated, all it took was for me to switch the focus!? Out loud, I said, "You're kidding."

I went and grabbed the other one and realized it had a focus twist on it too. I spent so much energy blaming the companies and their inability to make a cool, cheap toy that I didn't realize the answer was directly in front of me.

How often do we spend our day giving energy to outside sources without truly looking in? I was scrolling TikTok and a random video popped up and said, "When an eggshell is cracked from the outside, it is broken, when it's cracked from the inside, it is reborn." I blamed outside sources for the problem when I held the solution.

All that required me to fix the toys was to change my perspective and shift my focus. When Kambria and I do our daily affirmations, we are shifting our focus. We fill ourselves from within and connect to the Divine. We twist the knob to shift the focus from what the outside world says and turn inwards to fill our Divine spirits.

We can restore from the inside. Just speak to yourself like a two-year-old girl in the mirror! "I am strong! I am beautiful! I have a Divine purpose! I am a positive force for good! I am kind! I am happy!" Tell yourselves these things because they matter and will change how you view yourself.

I want to stand with everyone while looking in the mirror and tell them the positive affirmations they need to hear. But I can't do that. So, we need to do it. We must be the "Ryker," and lift our spiritual siblings!

As you strengthen yourself, you will be a beacon to those around you. You may not believe all the affirmations today, tomorrow, or anytime soon, but I promise that as you do them, the Universe will help you feel their truth one day.

There are mornings when I genuinely don't want to do affirmations, but my friend taught me a powerful practice that helps. I have a specific mirror where I do my affirmations. On this mirror, I write affirmations about myself. Keep in mind that the affirmations don't have to be physical. They can be goals you want to achieve, a particular mindset you want to change, or personality traits. But having them written on a mirror I look at daily helps remind me of Divine truths.

Every day we get bombarded by the outside world telling us we aren't enough. But my friend, you are enough! That is why filling yourself from the inside is so necessary. Relying on the world to tell you your worth will only lead to disappointment and self-hatred.

Besides affirmations, there is a brilliant thing I have been doing for years, but I just learned that there is actual science behind it! Mel Robbins does an entire podcast on it, and has a book.[8] The power of a damn high-five!

I am part of a bowling league, and we meet once a week. The other day when we were bowling,

---

[8] Take Complete Control of Your Life by Using the High-Five Habit! Mel Robins

I got a strike and high-fived myself! One of the ladies said, "Did you just high-five yourself?" Then a girl named Brooke, one of my dearest friends, said, "She sure did!" She was my boss and has been one of my best friends for a long time, so she knows me well.

When I high-fived myself, the people around me were surprised, but not Brooke, because that behavior has become a part of my character. I do it a lot because it helps! Try it. Right now. High-five yourself! Seriously. Mel Robins has an entire podcast dedicated to the practice of high-fiving yourself. It is titled *The One Science-Backed Habit You Need In 2023*. She also has a book called *The High Five Habit*. It will change your life. One morning after you high-five yourself, self-love will just click.

She specifically talks about creating a morning habit where you high-five yourself in the mirror after you brush your teeth! She calls this habit stacking, where you put a new habit along with a habit you are already doing. "As this practice is completed each day, you create a positive ripple effect in your life. You will improve your relationship with yourself. It is the secret to self-acceptance and self-love."

I strongly recommend listening to this podcast. Mel Robins continues to discuss the science behind high-fiving yourself and that in less than five days, you will see a drastic change in how you see yourself.

High-fives have been linked to improving motivation and performance in various activities.

Several studies with sports teams have been done.[9] They keep track of basketball players either high-fiving or knuckle bumping. The teams with the highest number of touches had higher statistics in their playing. The passing, the pick setting, and teamwork were overall higher. These simple team interactions improved their overall performance!

With the countless studies on the simple gesture of a high five, I recommend you start today. Right now. Just high-five yourself. It doesn't even have to be in the mirror! I do a high clap by my head and say high five!

I have been doing the high-five practice now for a while. Every day in the morning, I brush my teeth and high-five myself. This has created an energy of love towards myself. I don't look in the mirror and hate who I see. The woman standing in front of the mirror and the woman in the mirror are separate beings. I talk to the woman in the mirror with a kindness I never had before. I see her hurt, I see her heartache, I see her flaws, and I choose to love her.

Choosing to love myself became more manageable when I started high-fiving myself in the mirror in the mornings. Mornings have become my hardest but most sacred moments. Life has been a lot of shit lately. When I wake up, my stomach is full of anxiety, to the point where I throw up if I don't immediately invite peace to my morning.

9 Fournier, Julie. "High Five: An MVP Move." Ball is Psych, February 4, 2019.

That is why high-fiving myself has become such a powerful tool because it allows me to release that anxiety and do something that has been wired in my brain to raise my vibration.

If the high five isn't enough, I give myself a beautiful pep-talk. I speak to myself as I would my best friend. Acknowledging the woman in front of me as a divine soul has allowed me to shift my perspective of how I see myself. I see myself through the divine lens of infinite love.

Finally, I have fist-bumped the Universe. This one is fun because it helps me uniquely connect to my Divine. When I fist-bump the Universe, I acknowledge the unlimited Divine power we can access. I am creating space for an attitude of gratitude.

> I see her hurt, I see her heartache, I see her flaws, and I choose to love her.

Shifting your energy starts by creating habits that bring love into your life. These simple gestures may seem silly or awkward initially, but I have noticed a difference in my attitude and daily life! So, try it! What do you have to lose?

I had someone who I considered one of my dearest friends tell me that they didn't want me in their life. This was different than the one from earlier in this book, but they were very close together, time-wise! It seemed out of nowhere, and I was shocked and sad. I had bowling league right after this conversation, and I didn't want negative energy to ruin the night. I am at the point where if people don't want me in their lives, I won't fight or beg them. So, I was okay with letting her go, but I was still distraught and needed to switch my negative energy.

My dear friend and fellow bowler Pam Nebeker-Tolman is a Reiki master, does tapping therapy, and has many certifications in energy work.

When we were bowling, I asked her to help me release that negative energy because I wanted to enjoy the evening. She and I sat in the middle of the bowling alley, with me crying and us doing various tapping exercises.

Together, we were able to help me realign from within and connect to my Divine by recognizing that I am enough. We did this exercise for less than 10 minutes, and the tapping completely changed my energy. I released the chains of another person's decision and chose to recognize that I love and value myself.

I have spent so much energy reminding myself daily that I love myself. So, when other people make it abundantly clear that they don't love me, that is okay! My self-worth doesn't come from the love and acceptance that others give me!

My self-worth comes from connecting to my Divine and doing exercises that invite light and positivity into my life. I challenge you to take a step today to show yourself some love. Whether writing on your mirror, saying affirmations, doing a self-love meditation, giving yourself a high-five, or watching a tapping video on YouTube, you have many options! All you have to do is take that first step.

Chapter 9

Start Reframing

I have a circle of close best friends, all filling different roles in my life. One of my best friend's name is Haeli. If you don't have a Haeli in your life, manifest one! We have been best friends for over two years, and when we met, she was an instant best friend. Haeli is a life coach, therapist, and yoga teacher. She has been someone I look up to since day one.

Throughout our friendship, Haeli helped me accept and love my true self. I tend to be extremely harsh on myself, but Haeli has taught me the necessity of restructuring our thoughts. We were talking through some challenging things recently, and she mentioned that because I grew up without a mom, that probably makes me a spectacular mom.

The thoughts that went through my head were entirely negative. I told her I was not a very good mom. Then I listed the reasons why I wasn't a good mom. Her response was, "Or is the mom that beats her kids, mindfucks them, abandons them, or lets their boyfriend rape them the shitty-ass moms?"

As a therapist, she hears the darkest stories people hold within themselves, so my response didn't surprise her. I told Haeli she didn't always need to defend me. But she wasn't necessarily defending me; she was helping me reconstruct and reframe my thoughts.

Reframing how we speak to ourselves is essential. Speaking kindly to yourself is essential because your relationship with yourself is the most important one. Having a good relationship with yourself is the foundation of having good relationships with others. When you see and love yourself through the Divine lens of love, you can see others through that same unconditional love.

Reframing is a powerful tool when it comes to suicidal ideation. You are not a burden. You are a blessing. What are the thoughts you can focus on reframing today?

I have another tool you can add to your tool-belt if it feels right. The power of a cold shower! Cold water sounds horrendous, I am well aware! I turn on the shower warm, and then once I am in, I switch it to cold. While in the shower, I repeat affirmations that I need to work on believing. The one I have focused on most recently is "I am a good mom. I am a safe space for my children."

I repeat these affirmations because I have a core belief that I am not a good mom. My depression makes it difficult to have the motivation to be the peppy, happy teacher and mom I would like to be all the time. As I consistently utilize the tools I am learning, I can reconstruct my negative belief systems of not being the perfect mom.

Cold showers are not easy, but as I focus on saying affirmations that uplift and strengthen me, I am reminded of how strong I am. If I don't shower in the morning and have an off day, I can take a cold shower in the afternoon, which will change my mood. I am not a scientist, but I know studies are backing up the positive effect cold water has on your body.

> Speaking kindly to yourself is essential because your relationship with yourself is the most important one.

Focusing on the affirmations helps me realign my focus toward the Divine. Reshifting our focus truly comes down to the thoughts we allow in our minds and the words that come out of our mouths. I love Haeli, but she can't always be there to help me reconstruct my thoughts. I have to step into my power and say, "Enough is enough! I am fantastic, and no one else will tell me otherwise!"

Remember, the key to self-love is shifting our focus inward. Remember earlier when I talked about the knob on the storytelling projector for my phone? Having more self-love can be a simple fix, but you must know what to do. Saying affirmations, and high-fiving yourself, are seemingly small things that will help us shift our focus each day.

Take that first step to re-shift your focus and align it with the infinite love of the Universe. It may be as simple as twisting a little knob you didn't know was there to correct the focus! Shift your focus, and realign it with your Divine because you, my dear, deserve to see yourself through the lens of infinite grace and love.

My kids and I started a new bedtime tradition. Every night before bedtime, we cuddle and talk about our "Happy Highlights." I ask them three questions for the Happy Highlights. The first question is, "What made you smile today?" Second, "When did you have the opportunity to show kindness to another person?" Third, "When did you have the opportunity to show kindness to yourself?"

I created this nightly questionnaire because my son had been focusing on the negativity around him. One night, we were just talking (remember he is only four), and he kept repeating the same story of negativity that happened. It was important for me to validate his frustrations from the story, but I wanted him to move past them so he could see the positive things from his story.

Remember, life is about shifting our focus and moving the knob on the little projector just a little to see things more clearly. I asked what made him smile that day. This exercise is powerful because he actively thinks about things that make him smile throughout the day. Giving him an active goal to look for things that make him smile throughout the day will cause him to seek positive feelings.

Smiling causes your brain to release tiny molecules called neuropeptides.[10] These neuropeptides help fight off stress, reduce blood pressure, and release dopamine, serotonin, and endorphins. The Happy Highlights is a nightly reminder to look at things positively throughout the day because we see what we look for.

The second question I ask is if he had the opportunity to show someone else kindness. I phrase it like this for a couple of reasons. When we have the opportunity to show someone else kindness, do we take it? Or do we choose not to? This will open the conversation to why or why not he took the opportunity to help. The dialogue will then help him to reflect on his intentions behind things and not judge others for helping or not helping.

Divine insight can come from this question. Practicing the act of kindness can build a love for those around him. As he practices kindness, he will see people through unconditional love because one's ego and kindness to others can't coexist.

He won't always choose kindness, which is okay because none of us are perfect. We are practicing. I want to help him overcome his ego and seek opportunities to serve.

---

[10] "The Real Health Benefits of Smiling and Laughing." The Real Health Benefits of Smiling and Laughing | SCL Health, 2018.

Eventually, my son asked me the same questions. Answering those questions provided me with the opportunity to reflect on my day. It was fantastic that we both had an opportunity to remember and share our experiences of kindness.

The third question hits me hard. Did I have the opportunity to show myself kindness? I stop and think about if I have shown myself sincere kindness. For example, I might say "I went on two walks today, which were acts of kindness. I experienced nature and moved my body." Those are acts of kindness to yourself!

There are so many ways to show kindness to yourself. When I am working out, I started using aggressive self-love. During an exercise I struggle with, I start saying, "I am a badass! I am so amazing at everything I do! I can do hard things! I bet my ass looks amazing! These arms are sexy AF!" I just pump myself up!

The goal in life is to experience joy! Some of these tools we use for our mental health may seem silly, but why the hell not? What is stopping you from being silly and enjoying your life? Complimenting yourself? Do little things that give you small bursts of joy. You have to start somewhere.

I just started saying the most random, uplifting things to myself, and it was empowering! I was being a cheerleader and pumping myself up! Because, girl, why the fuck not?!

You are fucking spectacular, and you deserve to see yourself as the badass you are! So instead of saying something mean in your head, say something nice! Take the opportunity to show yourself kindness, do something for you. Instead of scrolling social media for 15 minutes, go for a walk.

I may be unable to ask you these three questions that I ask my son, but find someone who can be your Happy Highlight buddy! Have an accountability friend with whom you feel safe talking about these questions.

Even if that buddy is you in the mirror, ask these questions daily. You will see a positive shift in your mental health! Trust the Universe, and trust the positivity that surrounds you. You deserve to see your life through the divine lens of infinite and unconditional love. Just remember to do things that actively shift your focus and twist that knob.

Chapter 10

Light Overwhelms Darkness

In Winter of 2021, my husband and I started snowshoeing! It has quickly become a favorite date night of ours. We live in the middle of nowhere in Wyoming. We live on 400+ acres, so there are many places to explore!

On our first night of snowshoeing, the primary source of light we had was the moon. Our first goal was to get to a gate across a field that led to the river, but it's hard to see through the darkness when you lack light.

Our end goal was to snowshoe half a mile to the river. We tried to find the gate to the river as we walked through the darkness. But we weren't able to find the gate. When you rely solely on the dark to guide you, it is easy to get lost. We kept zigzagging and thought we were going in the right direction multiple times. We decided to turn around and head home. We could see our big barn with the outdoor light shining when we turned around.

It was simple to follow the light and make our way back home.

When we got closer to the barn light, other lights around the property began to fill the darkness. If I turned back to look at the darkness, I could still see it, but it no longer enveloped me. I was in the light; therefore, the light became part of me.

Darkness cannot lead you to your highest vibration of living. Whatever darkness may be weighing you down, it is time to release it. This is where more shadow work comes in. Dig deep into the darkness to discover the light.

As we fill ourselves with light, we can no longer get sucked into the lower vibration of darkness. We become light and shine a light on those around us. We can still see the darkness if we look back, but we are so full of light that we shine.

I have mentioned previously that I am a dog groomer. You see, I don't love dog grooming. It is not my passion. But right now, financially, it is a necessity. It supports my family and allows us to live financially stable lives. So often, I have told my husband how much I dislike it and don't want to do it.

While grooming last week, I listened to a live Q&A with Gabby. A woman asked how to reframe her mindset around her job because she hated it. Gabby talked about joy and the importance of making joy our goal. If your goal is to experience joy, you can't fail. I understand being happy is easier said than done.

If our goal is joy, we can't fail. When I heard this, I decided to change my mindset about grooming! I started listing things out loud that I love about grooming. I love dogs. My love for dogs borders obsession! When I see a dog, I always ask the owner if I can pet it (unless it is a working dog). Dogs are beautiful, kind, and loving. They are trusting and willing to learn. All dogs want to do is love.

When I am grooming dogs, I get to meet so many dogs! I help them feel better by removing mats and cleaning them up. I love helping them feel safe when I teach them how to relax around the new tools I use. Once, I had a dog terrified of the blow dryer and continuously bit at the dryer. But through softly spoken words, placement of the dryer, and confidence within myself, I could thoroughly blow dry that dog without her trying to bite the dryer. I focus on keeping positive energy flowing through me, and into the dogs. It is almost a meditative state for me.

I also love that this is a unique talent and skill. I love knowing how to shape a dog's face to fit the body shape. I experience joy when I finish a groom and see how beautiful the dog looks.

This week, a client called me later to thank me for doing her dog. She said he had never felt so soft and fluffy and that she would have to bring him back every couple of months. I feel joy when

I know my clients are happy because my ultimate goal is to feel joy and help those around me feel joy.

A client asked me why I could do her dog when so many groomers had failed before me. I told her it was all about our energy. When I have an anxious dog, I play relaxing frequencies. I breathe into my own peaceful state of mind and allow the dog to feel that peace. I find joy in the moment with each dog and allow the peace of our coexistence to be the energy that fills the room.

Choosing to have peace when I groom has been a process. If you are in an environment you dislike, change it. I don't specifically love grooming, but I love that I can feel peace and joy while working at a job that isn't my dream.

So, my friend, you may hate your job or life, but I challenge you to find something within that darkness that helps you feel joy. Today, make your goal joy, and you will not fail!

Some weeks I struggle deeply with depression. My depressive monster comes back into the room, and I can't get depression out. As a result, I half-assed my self-care and meditation time. I often want my depression to be gone, but I don't truly focus on things that bring light and love into my life.

Usually, when my depression knocks on the door, I can acknowledge her, do shadow work, and send her on her way. When I focus on fulfilling myself inwardly and connecting to the Universe, it is easy to ask the depression to leave because I am filled with light. But if I am not doing things to care for myself and connect with the Divine, I snowshoe backward into that darkness.

Our brains are a powerful tool. What we see depends mainly on what we look for. When I am constantly thinking about depression and finding a way out of it, I will be bound by it. That is why committing to joy is essential! When I am focused on seeing the joy daily, I will experience it!

Every day I have a choice to recommit to joy instead of sitting in my depression. It isn't always an easy choice, but as I focus on the Universe and the infinite love that has been given to me, I can experience true joy daily.

So, commit to joy! Make a promise to yourself that each day you will commit to joy! I have written down three ways for me to commit to joy daily. I didn't want to overwhelm myself by committing too much, so I have three daily promises I commit to in order to feel joy.

First, I promise to do morning meditations daily! The second promise is to dance every day! Thirdly I promise to actively look for things throughout the day that make me smile.

The first promise is to do morning meditations! Meditating and connecting to the Universe can ensure my focus is on goodness and light each day.

I want joy to begin with me. My depression is welcome to visit, but my goal is joy. The goal isn't to suppress the depression but to understand why those feelings are coming up and work through them. By doing so, we allow light to be our guide.

Seeing the depressive darkness doesn't mean it overwhelms you and suffocates you. There may be days when you feel like all you can do is get up to go to the bathroom. If that is where you are, acknowledge that and grow from it. Sit in the darkness for a day but don't let it overcome your entire life. What is something each day that can bring light into your life? One day it may be brushing your teeth, and another may be writing an entire book!

Don't judge yourself by the brightness of your light. It is about the growth of the journey, and some days we just don't have the brightest light. That is fucking okay. Own the ground you stand on because the darkness or light you feel is valid.

I choose to snowshoe in the light and acknowledge depression on her way. Joy begins with me. It doesn't matter what is happening around me because I choose to stay in the light! I am an infinite being experiencing the highest vibration of love and joy. My goal is to live at my highest vibration of joy and love, while also recognizing that life isn't always rainbows and unicorns shitting cupcakes.

Each day as I actively meditate, reframe thoughts and put effort into experiencing joy, my depression disappears. As I choose to see joy, I feel it and truly believe it. I believe joy begins with me, so whatever darkness or depression surrounds me, I can't walk into the abyss.

If joy begins with us, we need to commit to that joy. What are three acts of commitment to joy you can do daily to fill your soul? My first act is to meditate daily. As I meditate, I quiet the world around me. It is impossible to feel peace in chaos. My friend, focus today on joy and healing. When connected to the Divine, you can live on the highest vibration of love. By embracing your darkness and becoming light, you heal the world.

My second promise of commitment to joy each day is to dance! Dance with my kids in my kitchen, dance while doing chores, and just dance at any opportunity! There is an immense joy I experience when I choose to let go and move my body. I am not a graceful or talented dancer, but I enjoy it, and it brings more light into my life! Every day I dance because joy begins with me, and dancing brings me joy!

My third daily commitment is to actively look for five things that make me smile throughout the day. Five may be a stretch depending on my mental capacity, but there is always at least one thing in a day that makes me smile.

My family and I had the opportunity to attend Disney On Ice. It was a magical event! The characters were phenomenal, but the cameraman was my favorite person to watch. We were right next to him, and he made the show! His smile is permanently etched into my memory!

Every time I looked over at him, he had the biggest smile on his face. He was singing and genuinely seemed to enjoy his job. After the event ended,

I went to him and told him he had made the show because he had a smile on his face the whole time. He laughed and said he definitely enjoyed his job.

This man set a beautiful example of enjoying what we do. Whether or not that was his dream job, he enjoyed every moment. He made joy his goal. So often, I catch myself getting caught up in getting frustrated with the little things, and I forget to enjoy what is happening now. I stress about the future or worry about the past when I should focus on enjoying the moment and smiling through the show called Life.

Even in the darkest times, as you search for reasons to smile, you will find it. One of my favorite quotes is, "Light can be seen in the darkest of places if one only remembers to turn on the light." -Albus Dumbledore

What we focus on is what we see. The Baader Meinhof Phenomenon is a phenomenon that occurs when we start to see something that we previously overlooked. For example, when I need a sign from the Universe, I see Sunflowers everywhere. I notice them scrolling online, or I see bumper stickers with Sunflowers. But once I have thought about Sunflowers, I actively see them everywhere.

It is the same concept when you want to buy a new car. If you want a red car, all of a sudden, you will start noticing every time you see a red car. Your brain is actively looking for the object you are seeking.

This concept is also known as the frequency illusion. This term was coined in 2005 by a Stanford Linguistics professor named Arnold Zwicky.[11] What we focus on is what we see. This concept is critical to understand because when we focus on joy, that becomes what we see most often.

> "Light can be seen in the darkest of places if one only remembers to turn on the light."
> -Albus Dumbledore

As I commit to my daily acts of joy, I will experience joy in times of struggle because I am focused on joy. That is why my third commitment of finding five things throughout the day that made me smile is essential to my mental health. I seek joy regardless of what is going on in my day. Even if the most I can do that day is brush my teeth, I still seek joy.

Let's do an exercise together to focus on what is thriving in your life! This exercise uses mantras and mudras. Mantras are words or phrases repeated to oneself in rhythm with breathing. A mudra is the use of hands to focus on the brain. I love this tool because it uses both mantras and mudras.

Counting the numbers on my fingers is an example of a mudra. I touch my thumb to each finger while repeating the different phrases.

---

[11] Zwicky, Arnold M. "Why Are We so Illuded? - Stanford University." Standford.edu, 2006.

Instead of using the numbers, try saying these mantras combined with the mudra finger movement: "Joy begins with me. Peace begins with me. Joy is life's purpose. I experience joy daily. Joy is my goal. The Universe gives infinite light. I receive the Universe's light. I choose daily transformation. I choose daily truth. I choose daily light. I feel infinite love." As you practice these, you are actively inviting peace into your energy.

I recently listened to *Sail Away* by Lovelytheband. One set of lyrics says, "The past was only practice." This is so true! Every day is a new day and a new chance to change! Forgiveness is one of the greatest gifts you can give to yourself! You aren't meant to be perfect, and that is okay. You are meant to experience joy! Remember you can't guilt or hate yourself into growth and perfection. You can only love yourself into change.

Release the past, and choose today to make joy your goal. Commit to it. As we embrace the light and release darkness, we reprogram our DNA daily. We must work on our inner development to establish a conscious communication with that DNA. I can't just expect my depression to disappear. I have to replace it with positive and loving energy consciously. Doing mantras, looking for angel numbers, seeking reasons to feel joy, all of those exercises are ways to reprogram our neuropathways.

So my dear friend, if you are struggling, there is light to be held. If you are lost, find things today that can bring joy. Three things. Just pick three things today that you can commit to feeling joyful. You are worthy and deserving of light. If you feel trapped in the darkness, know you aren't alone and that you can experience light and joy.

It can be scary to say goodbye to the darkness, but fear doesn't control your life. You are in control. Trust the Universe and release the fear that binds you. We can manifest happiness and live joyfully, no matter the state of our mental health. Life is meant to be enjoyed, not just endured!

Choose today, my friend. You deserve all the joy in the world. What three things can you change today to commit to joy?

Chapter 11

Love The Little You

When I was four years old, I had a couple of dreams of my deceased mother. One of them was my dad, my grandma, and me, all standing in my parent's room holding hands. My mom was lying on the bed, and I saw her spirit float out of her body and go up through the ceiling.

This dream is significant because, as a four-year-old, I finally understood what was happening. The most remarkable analogy I have heard of a child losing a parent is this: a child and a parent are playing ball in the hallway, but the ball goes into a bedroom. The child retrieves the ball, and when they return, their parent is gone. They don't know where their parents went; they just vanished. The child is left wondering why the parent is no longer playing ball in the hallway.

Now that I have two children, I recognize the significance of a parent's role, which makes this analogy much more powerful. Because I hypothetically went into the other room to retrieve the ball and my mom vanished, my dream became momentous because I understood. I understood that my mom was gone, and she wasn't physically coming back.

The following dream is a "core memory" I have also held onto. I was on my mom's back, and we were running through a maze of flowers. The vision of that maze takes my breath away. When we exited the maze, there was a spectacular dock surrounded by the most vibrant, colorful flowers imaginable. We stood on the dock holding hands.

This place is named Kami Lake and has become the happy place I frequently visit during meditation. It isn't a real place, but the place I named within my dream. This dream taught me that I am not alone. I can always find peace in times of turmoil because Kami Lake is a state of mind, and I can always visit. Meditation has been a powerful gift of healing that I use frequently. There is a sacredness to having a meditative place to visit.

Have you ever had someone ask you what your happy place is? Kami Lake is my happy place. Identify a happy place for yourself if you have not already. Allow that to be a place of serenity that you visit. Create a place in your mind where your meditation self takes you.

When I was young, around four years old, I would smack my head on the concrete. This is something that I can't believe I am writing in my book. It seems humiliating that I would do that to myself. But I was a hurt little girl unsure of how to express her emotions. My mom was gone, and I didn't realize a mom's significance in life until I became one. My son is the age I was when I remember going and hitting my head on the concrete. The immense emotions it would take him to do that are overwhelming, and breaks my mama heart.

I have been working with a therapist who has helped me see that many of my adult actions are because of the unhealed trauma I experienced from my mom dying when I was that young.

As I connect to my inner child at Kami Lake, I see her and validate those emotions. Anger is a secondary emotion I deal with, but digging deeper to discover the hurt has brought immense healing. Little four-year-old Jamie didn't know how to express or healthily feel her feelings, so she would hit her head on the concrete. Now, as an adult, I strive to heal her every day. But anger is an emotion that bubbles up, and sometimes I am back to being that little girl hitting her head against the concrete.

It is all about rewiring and expanding my emotional tool belt. Rewiring is necessary as an adult because our brains are 90% developed by age five. Childhood trauma can affect attachment, physical health, emotional regulation, dissociation, cognitive ability, self-concept, and behavioral control.

I am not a neurologist or psychologist, but I have done my best to try to understand and heal my trauma. I still have a long way to go, but recognizing that healing needs to take place and then taking the necessary steps to experience that healing is key. We can't heal what we don't acknowledge.

Meditating with the dream of my mom carrying me at Kami Lake has brought immense healing. Through that, I can connect to my mother on a deeper level. We can connect energetically, and I go to her often when I need peace or answers.

This may sound like the most hippy-dippy shit, but healing is all about finding what works for us. You may be thinking, "This chick is fucking crazy. She has attempted suicide and meditates at a pretend, weird-ass lake." But you know what, my dear? Life is all about the journey. We can't expect others to fill our cup, we have to fill it ourselves. If we don't, we will forever be stuck as that damaged little child. I choose to heal her, I choose to love her.

Those dreams have been a guide for me to understand the Divine. I learned where my mom went and that she is safe and happy. My mom's energy surrounds me, and I can experience emotional healing. As I focus on the abundant love of her energy, I can release the hurt of that little girl. I release the anger that comes up and choose to feel the hurt behind the anger.

We get to choose to stay in our trauma or move past it. Don't stay silent. Get the help you need, and let's move through your trauma. Your inner child deserves healing and love.

We can't heal what we don't acknowledge.

What is an action you can do that will help you heal your inner child? I love my dance parties, I feel silly, and truly don't give a shit what I look like. Can I actually dance? Not really, but I can move! Do I look graceful doing it? No. But doing so helps me connect to little Jamie and let her know that it is okay to just exist, and that she is safe in her existence. So, what is your action to connect to your inner child?

Chapter 12

Choose Your Hard

Choose your hard! I came up with the saying when one of my best friends was going through a divorce. She was separated from her spouse and knew her marriage was over. She just didn't know how to pull the trigger for the divorce.

I have seen my sister go through a divorce, and I wouldn't wish that pain on anyone. I have seen the darkness and depth that experience gives. The growth my sister went through after her divorce is simply beautiful. So though that experience was filled with more pain than my sister has ever experienced, she grew into the person she needed to become.

I had told my best friend this, but the saying "Choose your hard" kept coming up. Getting a divorce is hard. Staying with someone when there is no real future is hard as well. She had to choose the hard she wanted to experience.

In my personal life, I hold on to that saying. Because as much as we wish it were, life isn't always full of unicorns and rainbows.

I first heard the story of Mohini, the tiger, in the book *Radical Acceptance* by Tara Brach.[12] Please do yourself a favor and listen to or read that book! It is also a tool I have used to see myself through the Divine lens of infinite and unconditional love.

In her book, she talks about Mohini the tiger. This tiger is a beautiful example of choosing our hard. The tiger spent most of her life in a 12x12 concrete cage with bars in the Washington Zoo. Passersby could see her anxiety because Mohini would pace back and forth. She walked a figure 8 pattern in her cage all day, every day.

The zoo built her a massive outdoor wildlife park with hills, ponds, and trees, similar to her natural habitat. Instead of exploring the park, she secluded herself in the corner and made a figure 8 path in a 12x12 space. She limited herself to that corner because that was the "hard" she knew. It would've been hard and scary to explore, but the beauty she could've experienced was phenomenal.

Mohini chose her hard, and that was spending the rest of her life in a limited corner. She missed out on so many spectacular experiences in life because she was afraid.

---

[12] Brach, Tara. *Radical acceptance: Embracing your life with the heart of a buddha*. New York, NY: Bantam Books, 2004.

I struggle deeply with eating and my health. I have worked with a doctor who tested me for various things. It turns out I have an autoimmune disease. I am not surprised, because my sisters do as well. Our mom having Lupus gave us a greater chance to have something.

Through the testing the doctor gave me, he gave me a list of about 20-30 things I can eat. My body reacts if I eat things that aren't on that list. The white blood cells go to fight, so I am nearly always congested. The first line of defense is your nasal passage. I can't "cheat" because the white blood cells react to everything.

Right now, my body can't handle black pepper. The white blood cells react to that negatively. Isn't that crazy? Something as simple as black pepper is an ingredient my body currently can't handle. I am continuously getting sick. Last night, I woke up and had to sleep with a bowl next to me in case I couldn't make it to the toilet.

I am supposed to eat like this for six months straight. Then, we can wean back in various types of food. We just have to give my body time to heal and restart.

I am so fucking sick of being stuck in my Figure 8! I am Mohini making circles of an unhealthy life, and I don't need to live like that. I don't need to wake up at 2:00 am to swallow, throw up in my mouth and have my husband stay home from work because I don't know if I can function the next day.

Yes, it will be hard not to go out to eat or to be extremely particular in how I prepare my food. But damnit, I am done being sick all the time. We choose our hard.

I love myself unconditionally, and because of that, I am willing to show my body that I will take care of her. I will choose my hard, knowing the Universe will support me. The Universe supports you too, my friend. So today, will you commit to a new hard for me? If you feel stuck in your figure 8, what can you change so you can see all the beauties life has to offer?

The goal is to finally see ourselves through the Divine lens of infinite unconditional love. I am not telling you to get a divorce or change your eating habits. But every day we get to choose our hard. Mohini is a devastating example of limiting ourselves because we fear what may be on the other side. But what if the other side is the most growth and beauty you can imagine?

My sister didn't know that her divorce would be the domino effect that changed her into one of the most loving and influential people I know. She did immense spiritual and self-healing. Her partner did immense healing as well. Years later, they are back together and are both in beautiful places on their journey. They both experienced darkness to achieve growth. Their divorce wasn't easy, but now they are two of the strongest women I know.

My sister, Allie, has spent the last six years being a full-time blogger. Before she started blogging full-time, she was at a crossroads with a job. She could continue working a 9-5 job or step into her dream of full-time blogging. She chose to begin a full-time blogging career. She spent 8-12 hours a day working on her blog. She didn't know shit about blogging, but gave herself a master's degree in blogging because she spent so much time learning.

She would tell me about the days that were so exhausting mentally that she wanted to quit. Some days she spent the entire day working on one portion of her blog. That shit wasn't easy! She wanted to give up so often! But instead of quitting, she persevered. She knew there were trees, hills, and ponds beyond the frustrations of her figure 8.

There were days when I would go over to her house in the late afternoon, and she would be sitting there with a messy bun, in sweats, with papers and her laptop sprawled out. I had no idea that a successful blogger didn't just sit down and write stories on a website. An extreme amount of work and time goes into building it.

She didn't know she would succeed with her blog the way she has, but every time she saw a new number rise or gain a new affiliate, she would share that success with us. We were cheering her on, even if we didn't see the shit behind the curtain or every time her website got hacked. She persevered through the hard, but she also knew we had her back and wanted her to succeed.

We have an infinite amount of spirit guides who have our backs and are cheering for every little success! Our family, our friends, and strangers on the street are cheering us on.

I didn't know all the struggles for Allie to build her blog, but I celebrated with her. Even if I didn't understand what she was talking about, I could share that excitement with her.

Her blog now brings in a six-figure income. She teaches others how to build their businesses through blogging and social media. My sister didn't know her blog would become a primary source of income, but she believed in herself enough to fight through the hard days.

She fought through the days that hackers stole her website, she fought the crashing of her website, and countless other struggles that I can't fully comprehend. She did all this because she saw herself through the Divine lens of infinite and unconditional love. She knew that her dream was worth fighting for because she was worth fighting for.

My sisters are vastly different in every aspect except for one—the diligence and willingness to believe in themselves because they know their worth. My sisters are older than me, so I truly get to see and follow the examples of my big sisters. They have stepped away from their figure 8 and now experience the beauties of the land.

Whether you are trying to be healthier, are experiencing the death of a relationship, or are trying to build a new career, you can do it. You can do hard things. You get to choose your hard because you control your destiny. You are not Mohini the tiger stuck in Figure 8 because you can choose to change. Is it hard to try something new or escape a toxic environment? Hell yes. But you deserve it.

There is so much light the world has to offer. So, my dear, what "hard" is holding you back? Choose today and pick a new hard because the growth you can experience is waiting for you to choose to step beyond that 12x12 cage you have created.

You get to choose your hard because you control your destiny.

Chapter 13
You Have A Toolbelt
For A Reason

Owning your inner power is your superpower.
When you look in the mirror, what do you
see? It may not always be who or what you want
to see, but a divine being is inside you waiting to
be unleashed.

At Estuary, I was painted by the beautiful
Carolyn Woods. We did a full body paint session.
She has competed in World of Body Paint and is an
all-around badass. I picked the theme Maleficent,
and she used my body as her canvas. It was magnificent. The empowerment I felt being painted,
and then photographed, was profound.

Miss Carolyn is amazing. She is like an adopted
mom, so being able to be painted by her was a
beautiful experience.

We went with a Maleficent theme because the
live-action movies are my favorite. The portrayal
of Maleficent is something I connect with on a

profound level. Maleficent is powerful and loves deeply. She isn't perfect, but defends her loves with her soul. She is beautiful on the outside but even more stunning on the inside.

Maleficent has become an emblem in my life. When darkness traps me, I remember that I am her. I am an icon of power, and there are no limitations in the Universe except the ones I place on myself. I am that badass bitch that defends her world against the negativity of the Universe.

We all have this powerful human inside of us. It is all about knowing your worth. I know I am not a woman the world can fuck with, because I strive daily to align my intentions with the Universe. I know my worth and the infinite love and power the Universe holds for me.

The more I get to know myself, the more I realize this powerful version of me is my alter-ego. Having an alter-ego has helped me connect to my divine by seeing my divine qualities. I see myself in Maleficent. To me, the name holds power and beauty.

When I look back and see the body-painted pictures, I see myself through the divine lens of abundant love. I am a powerful divine soul who can genuinely take on the world. We all have an alter ego that is a badass who can conquer anything! You just need the right tools to help you embrace your power because you control your destiny.

In Cohasset, Massachusetts, there is a Vedanta Centre. Their website describes the center as "a non-sectarian place of worship dedicated to all the religions of the world, where people of different faiths may come together and worship the One Spirit who is called by many names. Our philosophy is based on the universal teachings of Vedanta as expounded by India's 19th-century mystic and world teacher, Sri Ramakrishna. His chief disciple Swami Vivekananda brought Vedanta to the West in 1893."[13]

Every Sunday, Sudha Ma, the leader of the center, gives beautiful sermons. In one sermon, she talked about negativity and how you can physically flick out emotions that no longer serve you! Since she taught this tool, I have used it frequently! I physically flick emotions that no longer serve me. This is not to say I don't feel them. I simply choose to release the negativity of those feelings.

I don't slam my head into the concrete because I have healthy coping mechanisms. There are healthier ways to feel emotions than hurting ourselves.

There is a common saying that has become a grounding meditation that I often repeat. "A bad attitude is like a flat tire. You can't get very far until you change it." We must choose to release the negativity that binds us, or we will create a spiritual

---

[13] Maker, Site. "Vedanta Centre, Cohasset, MA, Spiritual Center, Meditation Classes, Vedanta Philosophy." Vedanta Centre, Cohasset, MA, spiritual center, meditation classes, Vedanta philosophy, 2020.

dam that will stunt our divine growth. It is hard to know how to grow if our only coping mechanism is to bang our heads against the concrete.

Learning tools that help rid ourselves of negative energy is critical to breaking down the dam. I have created a list that I call my transformation checklist.

Cher Lyn wrote in her Mystic Art Medicine Oracle Cards, "The power of Transformation lies in your ability to find the light within the shadow and make the connection, infusing focus on its light quality instead of the darkness. Everything you think, feel, and do creates lessons in your world. Inside you, great intelligence, wisdom, and love are ever-present. The beliefs you have been taught are the hindering factor here."[14]

"A bad attitude is like a flat tire. You can't get very far until you change it."

We have all the tools inside to transform negativity into positivity. I am grateful for my checklist because it reminds me that I have healthy ways of releasing anger. I don't need to take out my anger on myself or those around me.

My transformational list is: turning on music and dancing, meditating, flicking away anger, doing a plank/quick challenging exercise, listing

[14] Lyn, Cher. *Mystic Art Medicine Oracle Cards Tools for Transformation*. Sedona, AZ: Soyink, 2009.

three things I am grateful for, and using my thumb to pinky, thumb to ring finger, etc., to breathe and remember that peace begins with me. When I need to release anger, I also have a wall exercise. I push against a wall as hard as possible and let out the most ferocious growl ever. This may seem weird, but it helps release the anger!

I was experiencing big emotions, and my son could tell I was frustrated. He said, "Mom do you want to push against the wall and growl with me?" My five-year-old recognizes big emotions and has a toolbelt. It was a beautiful experience seeing him actively using those tools to help another person. Thank you, TikTok, for that healthy, anger-releasing tool!

All of these are means to create positivity where negativity exists. We don't need to slice our wrists or hit our heads. There are other ways to express and validate our emotions, my dear, I promise.

When it rains, look for rainbows; when it is dark, look for stars! There is always something positive we can find when looking for it. If we say life is so hard, everything is awful, and I hate XYZ; we are creating more of that low vibrational energy. As we actively strive to switch our mindset, we can create a positive environment that forges a life of beauty and love.

I challenge you to create your transformation list! What can you do when experiencing negative emotions and want to adjust them? It is okay to have anger appear, but what you choose to do with it will determine your Divine growth. Will we stay stuck hitting our heads against the concrete, or will we find healthy ways to express that powerful emotion? I choose to change. I choose positivity.

I refuse to be a negative light to my family and those around me. I will continue to work on myself and grow just a little each day. I know that through my connection with my Divine, I can feel infinite love because I am infinite. You are infinite, and there is abundant love that you can embrace and connect to every moment.

Chapter 14

About Damn Time

Y ou. This life is about you and your experience. Why waste it living inauthentically or spending time hating yourself? It doesn't make you happier to live inauthentically. Hating yourself creates unnecessary pain. So why, friend? In this book, we have talked about self-love tools and told stories about healing. But have you truly embraced the authentic you?

What does embracing the authentic you even mean? That is a question I can't answer for you, but I can tell you my answer. Let me first tell you a little more about me.

I was raised in a highly religious household. I was a "Latter-Day Saint," also known as Mormon. I was taught that you get married and have babies. When I was twelve, we did a youth activity where we wrote our "dream" man and all of the qualities we wanted him to possess. They had us keep the list as a reminder of "what we wanted." Activities like this and Sunday School lessons frequently taught that, as young women, we should want to get married in the temple and have an eternal family at any cost.

You can't know what you want or the kind of lifelong partner you want when you don't even know who you are. They teach you to hold onto the belief that a temple marriage is everything, and keeping that mindset for life is essential. By getting baptized at eight, I committed my life to a God and carried the guilt of not being perfect for Him.

Each of my family members had left the church by the time I was nineteen, except for me. I served an eighteen-month mission where you have no contact with your family outside of a once-a-week email. On this mission, you teach others about the church.

I was very devoted, but I hated myself. No matter how perfect I was, I was never enough. I tried to follow the rules. I repeatedly told myself that I wanted to get married in the temple and have babies. I had so thoroughly convinced myself this is what I wanted, because I believed in the church with my entire being.

So, I believed myself when I said I wanted an eternal marriage because that was all I knew. That was everything to me, but I had feelings for girls. I denied and suppressed these feelings. I had convinced myself that liking girls was a feeling that would pass. I wanted to follow God and do the "right" thing.

The church and extended family members told me that it was just a struggle, a trial from God. In the church, same-sex attraction is not a sin if you don't act on it. If you engage in a same-sex relationship, though, it is a sin.

When I was twenty-two, I met a wonderful man whom I still love dearly. He is my best friend. He loves me for me, even before I even knew who I was. We got married less than a year after we met, as was typical for Mormons.

The entire purpose of the Mormon religion is to have an eternal family, to be "sealed" in order to reach the highest Kingdom of God. I wanted to do the "right" thing, and never truly allowed myself to believe I was gay because that simply wasn't an option with my dedication to my religion. I believed in my religion more than I believed in myself. So, we got married, and had two beautiful children.

The Mormon Church teaches that all things are a trial of faith. So, though I "struggled" with liking girls, it was just a trial from God that I could overcome because of my commitment to Him. Now, looking back, I know it is a load of shit. My sexuality is not a trial of faith, or a test of loyalty to God. I don't love God more by suppressing a big part of me.

In 2021, when I left the church, I started to discover who I was. I learned how I connect to my divine; I learned what it means to be a divine soul; I learned true spirituality. I learned how to love myself. I released the guilt of not being perfect. It wasn't my job to bring my family back to the "fold of God." It was my job to love myself and accept who I am.

When I left the church, it was like a weight had been lifted off my chest. I no longer believed in a God that would make me one way but not expect me to live true to the way I was made. Healing after I left the church didn't happen overnight. It took me almost three years of self-discovery to realize I am worthy just as I am. As I healed the inner parts of my soul by shifting my perspective to see things through the Divine lens, I realized regardless of my sexual identity, I had been relying on another person to make me feel whole.

Acknowledging my sexual identity allowed me to look deeper into my relationship with my husband. I was unfulfilled because I was relying on him for my happiness. It took a lot of shadow work to discover what I had buried so thoroughly. Myself. I thought by accepting that I am queer, getting a divorce, and living my life as a lesbian, I would be happier. That isn't the case at all. Whether or not I am a full lesbian, bi, pans, etc., is irrelevant because right now, I am choosing me. I am choosing to fall in love with myself.

I don't know what the future entails. All I know is for the first time in my life, I am choosing to love me. When I look in the mirror, I get excited to talk to myself. There is peace in releasing the expectation of gaining anything from other people. You make yourself whole. Throughout this process, I have learned that you can have the most fantastic human in your life, but no one else can heal your soul.

It took me a long time to understand why I had so much darkness. Growth is never overnight. We must be intentional about the life we want to live. I was just going day to day, hoping my mental health would get better. I had to drastically change my life to experience peace within. It all started with the way I look at myself.

Living an unfulfilled life was impacting my mental health and my ability to be a healthy human and the best mom I can be. We don't choose who we are. All you can do is love who you are, and do your best to be a good soul. Embrace your authenticity because that is the best thing you can offer the world.

Throughout this journey of self-healing, I have learned that it doesn't matter how much other people love you. If you don't love yourself, you will stay trapped in your own darkness. Falling in love with the life you live, begins by falling in love with who you are. I began to fall in love with who I am for the first time in my entire life.

When I told my husband that I liked girls, he already knew and loved me anyway. We stayed married; we loved each other. I wanted to *want* a life with him. I wanted to *want* all of him, but I can't give myself to someone entirely until I fully love myself.

Telling my husband that right now I can't invest in our relationship has been hard. Seeing my sexuality has taught me that sexuality is not a choice, and that it is hard too. There has been immense confusion when it comes to my sexuality, and I wouldn't choose that confusion if I could! But we can't live our lives in a way that denies our true happiness, and by ignoring a part of our identity, we choose not to love ourselves fully. I was standing in the way of my happiness because I was afraid to embrace who I am.

I didn't want to hurt Josh, I didn't want to take a step back from our relationship. We lived a good enough life. But I was tired of good enough. I thought our marriage was unfulfilled because I am gay, but I was just existing in a state of self-hatred, and that was why my life was unfulfilled. The reasoning behind my unhappy relationship was so much deeper than just my sexuality.

I was tired of having shitty mental health. It took me a year of true devotion to my spiritual healing journey and mental health to understand why my mental health was so fucked up. I was existing without intention, I was building a life that wasn't true to who I was because I didn't know who that was. I am a Divine Being that is a powerful source to be reckoned with. The negativities of the world can no longer overwhelm me.

So, I am taking the steps necessary to find healing because I love myself. Finally, after all this time, I can write in this book that I truly love myself. Having self-love hasn't instantly healed everything, and it genuinely takes effort to feel love daily for myself. But I am tired of hating myself, and I am tired of living a life where I am unfulfilled.

A partner can't fill your cup, my dear. If you aren't filling your cup, it will always feel empty regardless of your relationship status.

That is why being honest with yourself, loving yourself, and being kind to yourself matters because YOU matter. This life is about your experience, so why waste time living inauthentically or happy enough?

Did you know your brain doesn't know the difference between a lie and the truth? The brain simply believes things are real.[15] So, in your head, if you are constantly degrading yourself, your mind is going to believe it. You have to cut off the negative thoughts immediately. Your brain will believe what you tell it, and you create your reality by the thoughts you form.

Falling in love with yourself is a choice. One you have to make every day. When you wake up, are you choosing you? I look in the mirror and high-five myself every fucking day. I am my own best friend. I have given my power away to so many people. Best friends, Josh, even my kids. I am taking back my power. I will never give my power away again.

If giving your power away to others is something you struggle with, I recommend power posing. Stand up, feet shoulder width apart, put your hands on your hips, and say, "I am reclaiming my power!" Do it over and over until you feel the

---

15 Hamilton, David. "Does Your Brain Distinguish Real from Imaginary?" David R Hamilton PHD, August 9, 2022.

truth of that statement. You are reclaiming your power. No one can take that away from you, and no one has power over you.

What you see is what you get in this life. If you choose to be mean and degrade yourself, that is what you will see within yourself. If you choose to obliterate your self-worth each time you look in the mirror, there will be no self-esteem or self-compassion.

You have to start fighting for yourself. No one else will fight for your happiness as hard as you will fight for your happiness. So, stop accepting anything less than the ultimate self-love and compassion the abundant, infinite Universe offers.

Manifest the life you want for yourself. Someone told me a few weeks ago that they don't believe in manifestation. My response was blunt but accurate. Manifestation happens whether or not you believe in it. Simply put, they are the thoughts we form in our heads. Whether it is a passing thought of I am fat, or an in-depth meditation where you allow love and creativity to flow. All of these thoughts play a role in creating the life you are living, whether negative or positive.

The next book you should read is *The Law of Attraction* by Esther and Jerry Hicks. That book thoroughly talks about manifestation. I don't think we give our minds enough credit because, through intentional manifestation, we can create the life of our dreams. Your thoughts are the only Universal limitation.

If you tell yourself every day *I hate you, you're so ugly and fat, blah blah blah...* that is all you will believe. Every day, I tell myself I am a successful motivational speaker with multiple best-sellers. That is where I see my life, and as I continuously put that in the Universe, that is what is happening. I have a massive team behind me on this book, and it hasn't even been released.

We create our reality, starting with the thoughts we allow to preside in our minds. Each day, I take a few minutes and visualize my goals in life. I put energy into the things I want. Doing this is an intentional manifestation. My meditation corner has a poster board with my yearly goals. I spend time each day looking over these goals because I am the creator of my life.

Setting goals helps me find purpose in myself. When you set goals that you see every day, it keeps your mind focusing on your deepest desires. This allows you to start living for yourself because they are *your* dreams. This is your life. No one else's.

I have two beautiful children, and I have stayed alive for them. I lost my mom when I was two, and I have had to process healing for many years from her death. I will not do that to my children; I had to find a reason to live beyond just them. I had to look inward and face my demons to heal. The time spent in meditation or just sitting with myself has been a lot, and there were times when I wanted to look away. But the greatest gift we can give our children is our healing.

This book was almost called "Love Me Enough." After my September 2022 attempt, when I was at Estuary, I began learning that I had to love myself enough to live for myself. Yes, I adore my children and don't want them to suffer like I did from losing a parent, but that can't be my only reason for living.

By not healing the inner parts of my soul, I was heading toward a successful suicide. After multiple fucking attempts, something in my life had to change, and I had to be the one to change it. You choose your hard. Telling your partner you can't be a partner right now is hard. Living a partially fulfilled life is hard.

What do you want in your life? What will bring you happiness? What will lighten the darkness we carry? I saw a random quote on Facebook once that said, "The courage to leave behind what's not for you anymore is the same courage that will help you find your way to what is."

Life is scary; healing is scary. But we need to stop shrinking to fit places we have outgrown. As you live life intentionally, you can shapeshift your reality to create something more meaningful. We are creatures of habit, but you can shift yourself out of rigid patterns that limit the life you are meant to live. Doing this takes a conscious effort. You can't just slide into healing. You have to actively move toward it.

Choosing love is consciously found in the experience of every moment. You must choose to transform that which is in you. Allowing a transformation of self can set you free. Living 11+ is possible. If you want peace, the only functioning place to propagate peace is within your conscious mind by using an open heart. Lean into the practices we've talked about, and do the work. Healing is worth the work, my friend.

What you resist, persists. To reclaim your power, you must face what you have been neglecting. Have you done the meditation moments? Have you spoken kindly to yourself? Have you applied any of the tools we have talked about?

Spend quality time meditating and exploring the Universal void inside your soul. Look inward, and you will find healing. The Universe has unlimited resources to help you live the life you desire.

If you unknowingly suppress a painful experience, you will continue to re-create similar feelings to the original hurt. When similar patterns arise, it is our soul's way of getting us to look at the fucking darkness! Ask yourself, why does the same thing keep coming up?

I told my husband there was a reason my sexuality came up so frequently. It was because I buried that part of me, drastically affecting my mental health. But you can heal and find peace in your transformation.

I used to be afraid of the future because it was unknown. But the future is full of transformation and change! I believe transformation is laced with absolute magic. The Universe is divine and full of magical healing. Lean into the strength the Universe holds.

I was sitting at a bay in Oregon, writing in my journal. I wrote down words that I had been feeling for years. I grabbed those words off the paper and threw them into the ocean. I no longer needed to carry the burden of beliefs that no longer serve me. The Universe is strong enough to hold what no longer serves you; pass it along.

The kids and I came to visit my family in Oregon. We went to the beach, and I played with my kids. My son asked me to swim, and I have been trying to say yes to things with him more.

In my life, especially with my kids, I want to be more present, so I said yes. Loving myself authentically has given me the desire to be present. The water was cold, and I didn't go above knee level, but my kids kept running to me. I would chase them, and then they would run away. The ever-constant waves came back and forth as we played.

The tide must go out before it can come in. The same is true in life. Sometimes, we must let go of something before something more significant can occur. We must let go of feelings and pain that no longer serve us.

Courage isn't about not being afraid. Courage isn't the absence of fear because I am still afraid. Courage isn't a fearless state of mind, but as we train our minds, we can use courage as an action despite fear.

Allow fear to transform into faith in the Universe. You will have an abundant and fulfilled life, but you must take the steps. I must take the steps necessary to close this chapter of my life with my husband. Moving past our fears, we can intimately understand courage and gain a greater sense of peace.

The abundant peace I have felt with my decision to fall in love with myself is life-changing. We can't stunt our growth for other people. Peace comes from accepting who we are and loving ourselves anyway.

For me to release this book, I have to be authentic. If I am living a lie, I can't be authentic. The entire book would be pointless. In pouring my soul into others' lives, I was choosing inauthenticity because I loved them instead of me.

You can't force yourself to live a life never meant for you. Living your life for others isn't your purpose. The more I got to know myself authentically, the less I wanted to live the life I was living. I was living in a constant state of depression because I thought that it had to be that way. I thought since I had depression, I would always be depressed.

> Moving past our fears, we can intimately understand courage and gain a greater sense of peace.

The sense of peace I have felt since embracing myself as an infinite divine energy source has been immense. Finding my source of depression was in accepting who I am. Wanting to end my life isn't a desire I have anymore because I love myself enough to live for myself. I thought it would be easier on my kids and husband if I didn't exist. But really, I was afraid of stepping into what I truly am because I have to do it alone.

I can't rely on anyone else for my happiness. Something always kept me from loving myself and being truly happy. Finding healing took a lot of time, which is okay. You can't expect growth and healing overnight. The only one standing in the way of your inner peace is you.

No one spends as much time with you as you do. So, speak to yourself kindly, feed your soul, and love yourself. There is no reason to continue down a path of self-hatred and self-destruction. Embrace your inner power, connect to the Universe, and *choose* to heal.

I used to believe that people don't change. That statement no longer stands true to my beliefs. If we couldn't change, we wouldn't have a purpose. But you are worthy of change, and you are worthy of keeping promises to yourself. Promise today to be a safe space for everyone, including yourself.

You are worthy of self-love. You are worthy of living. You are safe here. Together we can de-stigmatize talking about suicide because we can fight the darkness. Brazilian Amazons use the term Haux Haux (pronounced Haush), meaning "I see your soul." It is a standard greeting of seeing someone as they truly are. I leave you with this, Haux Haux. You are not alone in this life. Silence equals suicide, and we are silent no more.

The Universe created you. This life was meant for you. Taking care of yourself, loving yourself, and embracing who you are isn't selfish. Self-care is not selfish! What is one thing in your life that you can change to live more authentically to yourself and love yourself more thoroughly? At the beginning of this chapter, I asked, have you embraced the authentic you? My answer is finally yes. What is your answer?

Extra Thanks...

I want to thank my publishing team for the immense work they have put into this book. Especially my editor, Chloie, for the countless times bouncing ideas back and forth, and for all the brilliant edits! Chloie, you are simply the best.

Printed in the USA
CPSIA information can be obtained
at www.ICGtesting.com
LVHW010532100924
790397LV00009B/168

9 798989 862504